THE SPANISH FLU

THE SAD STORY OF ONE OF THE WORST
GLOBAL PANDEMIC OF 1918

By

NATHAN GRISHAM

© Copyright 2020 by Nathan Grisham
All rights reserved.

This report is towards furnishing precise and solid data concerning the point and issue secured. The production was available with the possibility that the distributor isn't required to render bookkeeping, formally allowed, or something else, qualified administrations. On the off chance that exhortation is important, lawful, or proficient, a rehearsed individual in the calling ought to be requested.

The Declaration of Principles, which the American Bar Association Committee and the Publishers and Associations Committee have accepted and supported.

Not the slightest bit is it lawful to replicate, copy, or transmit any piece of this report in either electronic methods or the printed group. Recording of this distribution is carefully disallowed, and any capacity of this report isn't permitted except if with composed authorization from the distributor. All rights held.

The data given in this is expressed, to be honest, and predictable, in that any risk, as far as absentmindedness or something else, by any utilization or maltreatment of any approaches, procedures, or bearings contained inside is the singular and articulate obligation of the beneficiary per-user. By no means will any lawful obligation or fault be held against the distributor for any reparation, harms, or money related misfortune because of the data in this, either straightforwardly or by implication.

Particular creators claim all copyrights not held by the distributor.

The information in this book is offered for educational purposes exclusively and is all-inclusive as so. The introduction of the data is without a contract or any assurance confirmation.

The marks used shall be without consent, and the distribution of the mark shall be without the consent or support of the proprietor of the mark. All trademarks and trademarks within this book are just for explanation and are held clearly by the owners, who are not associated with this record.

Table of Contents

Introduction 1

What Is Flu (Influenza)? 3

Origin Of Influenza 20

Influenza Pandemics In History 26

Spanish Flu 33

History Of 1918 Spanish Flu 44

    Social Disruption And Public Health Lessons 54

    The Site Of Origin 57

How Do Viruses Cause Pandemics 62

    Discovery 63

    Structure 65

    Function 66

    New Discoveries 68

Why The Second Wave Of The 1918 Spanish Flu Was So Deadly . 70

    How The Spanish Flu Got Its Name 71

World War One's Role In The Worst Ever Flu Pandemic 76

The U.S. Military And The Influenza Pandemic Of 1918–1919 80

    Going To War 83

    A Lethal Virus 86

Influenza In The Camps 89

How The 1918 Pandemic Frayed Social Bonds: Story 95

Wear A Mask And Save Your Life: The 1918 Flu Pandemic 100

Analysis: Spanish Flu Pandemic Proves Social Distancing Works .. 103

Looking Back At The Laws That Came With The 1918 Spanish Flu Pandemic 106

Economic Effects Of The 1918 Influenza Pandemic 108

Stronger Pandemic Response Yields Better Economic Recovery 116

    Evaluating Economic Consequences 117

    Banking Issues 119

How The 1918 Flu Pandemic Revolutionized Public Health 121

Misconceptions About The 1918 Flu, The 'Greatest Pandemic In History' 126

Flu Pandemic Of 1918: 5 Lessons Taught 132

    Precautions 133

    Here And Now 133

    Shortages 134

How The 1918 Spanish Flu Pandemic Changed The Nursing Profession: An Interview 135

    How Did The Nursing Profession Change As A Result? 137

    The Health-Care Industry Overall Changed, As Well? 137

So The Spanish Flu Led To Changes In How We Respond To Disasters? 138

Even With All These Advances, What More Needs To Be Done? 139

8 Things To Know About Pandemic Influenza 141

Conclusion... 144

INTRODUCTION

Every winter, there is a persistent question people ask regarding influenza. Many citizens fear influenza for reasonable intentions, some fear unjustifiably because of insufficient awareness of flu epidemics such as the one in 1918. The rational concerns we have derived are from other groups' unique disadvantages, such as older persons, children, and pregnant women.

The unjustified concerns were focused on predictions of an influenza epidemic as devastating as the 1918 pandemic, during which more than 30 times as many influenza deaths occurred in the United States in a typical year. Around one in a hundred people died of influenza in 12 months.

Experts examined the shape of the two protein molecules which stick out of the influenza virus surface. Hemagglutinin is one protein that allows the virus to bind to our cells to be reached. The other is neuraminidase, which stops molecules of the flu virus from adhering to one another. If the influenza experts find a mixture of the same proteins as the 1918 pandemic virus strain, which is labeled H1N1, the alert is close.

The H1N1 virus is not new; it developed prior to 1976 and triggered a series of unpredictable incidents. If a substantial portion of the population has not been subjected to a common H1N1 virus, the

Introduction

risk for a worldwide influenza epidemic is especially great. Throughout 1976, influenza researchers became worried as they were entering a time where the type of immunity to H1N1 nearly vanished from the population.

Those that had been born and died as infants in 1918 were about 60 years old in 1976. Those under the age of sixty had no tolerance to the 1918 epidemic. The fear was heightened by the political forces who carried out a 'Swine flu' vaccine campaign, which affected only five hundred men, around twenty-five of whom died, and triggered a paralytic disease called the Guillain-Barre syndrome. The results of the system are impossible to quantify. Perhaps only a few lives from an epidemic of flu that was clearly burned out on its own were spared.

There was fair fear over an H1N1 virus pandemic, but there was no worry regarding a re-visit of a virus that might affect the 1918 influenza virus.

We see flu viruses with the mixture of H1N1, but with no particularly strong virulence. We won't see a recurrence of the sort of lethal pandemic that marked the pandemic of 1918.

The Spanish Flu

WHAT IS FLU (INFLUENZA)?

Grippe is a respiratory infection that attacks the mouth, nose, bronchi, and, occasionally, the lungs. Influenza viruses are distinct and develop and shift from year to year.

To certain individuals, illness is a drawback over a matter of days. For some, influenza may contribute to respiratory complications, medical stays, and even death. According to the World Health Organization (WHO), 5 to 10 percent of adults and 20 to 30 percent of children have flu per year, and 3 to 5 million of these cases are extreme, contributing to around 250,000 to 500,000 dead.

In the United States, the Centres for the Care and Prevention of Diseases (CDC) reported 80,000 fatalities and 900,000 hospital visits from flu during the 2017 to 2018 flu season to render it the deadliest flu season in at least four decades.

The Italian term 'influenza' simply means "effect," a term that Italians have used since at least the 1500s for sickness since, like many people, they assumed that, as the *Douglas Harper Etymology Dictionary* states, stars have an effect on wellbeing. Several significant influenza pandemics have existed throughout history. The 1918–1919 pandemic, recognized as the Great Pandemic, for example, affected 20-40% of the world's population, and the Centre for Disease Control and Prevention (CDC) reported 50 million people died as a consequence.

Often identified as "Spanish flu," the pandemic is thought to have originated from Spain.

Throughout 2009-2010, there was a more modern pandemic of a different version of the influenza virus H1N1. The infection is sometimes named "swine flu," since the strain is identical to a pig infection (not that it may be transmitted by swine or pork).

Around April 2009 and April 2010, the swine flu pandemic triggered an estimated 43 million to 89 million infections in the United States. The CDC reported H1N1-related deaths to be between 8,870 and 18,300 during this time.

Causes

The three major influenza virus forms that induce illness in humans are A, B, and C. Influenza A and B viruses cause severe illness epidemics in the United States nearly every year, while influenza C triggers only minor respiratory symptoms and is not thought to contribute to CDC epidemics. The influenza A virus is categorized into subtypes, and both A and B are graded as strains.

It is necessary to remember that although there are multiple forms of grippe, "stomach grippe" is not necessarily a form of influenza. This is gastroenteritis, a lining infection triggered by a virus, bacteria, or parasite.

Avian influenza (bird flu, H5N1) is also an influenza virus that usually impacts only humans. It is very rare for people to catch it, and only around 700 cases of this bird flu have been confirmed since 2003 by the CDC in 15 countries. It is typically transmitted exclusively by birds and generally does not propagate amongst humans as other influenza forms.

Another rare bird flu, dubbed H7N9, occurred in China in 2013 for the first time. Since then, the virus has triggered several hundred human infections annually in China; but from 2016 to 2017, there was an increase in cases when 766 people were registered in China. The H7N9 virus does not seem to propagate easily among individuals.

Like bird flu, influenza A and B viruses are very contagious and can be transmitted from person to person by the cough or sneeze of an infected person. In 2018, researchers reported that the virus can only transmitted by breathing microscopic particles called aerosols. Many studies have found that such contagious particles will fly up to six feet after a sick person exhales them.

Symptoms

The effects of the common cold and flu are sometimes combined. In fact, flu symptoms are more extreme than cold symptoms, based on the CDC, but it may be challenging to discern the difference between cold and flu. For, e.g., people with flu typically develop fever, whereas people with colds hardly develop a fever. Any more typical signs and symptoms of influenza are present here:

- headache
- aching muscles, especially in your back, arms, and legs
- fever
- chills and sweats
- sore throat
- dry, persistent cough
- weakness
- nasal congestion

Treatment

According to the WHO, most patients who become diagnosed with influenza recover within one or two weeks without medical attention. "Extensive time, adequate fluids, and appropriate rest are really necessary for someone who has an influenza infection in order to recover completely," said Dr. Susan Donelan, the medical director for health epidemiology at Stony Brook University, New York.

Over – the counter painkillers like ibuprofen (Advil, Motrin, etc.) and aspirin can help relieve discomfort and ease pains and aches during influenza. Decongestant drops and cough syrups also help to alleviate the symptoms, but always consult a physician before offering children an over-the-counter remedy.

Many patients are at greater risk of flu safety problems that may contribute to hospitalization or death. It covers individuals under 65, children under 5, pregnant women, and people with other types of health problems such as lung disease, asthma, renal failure, and diabetes.

In certain instances, even relatively safe people can get seriously ill with grip. Spanish flu, for instance, destroyed many generally stable people between 20 and 50 years of age. The explanation for the elevated mortality rate is still unclear among young adults.

According to the American College of Emergency Physicians, signs that show that influenza requires immediate care include the following:

- Difficulty breathing or shortness of breath.
- Chest pain or abdominal pain.
- Sudden dizziness.
- Confusion.
- Severe or persistent vomiting.
- Flu-like signs that tend to change then worsen with fever and cough.
- Swelling in the mouth or throat.

In children, emergency symptoms include:

- Fast breathing or trouble breathing.
- Bluish skin color.
- Not drinking enough fluids.
- Not waking up or not interacting.
- Being so irritable that the child does not want to be held.
- Flu-like effects that change and then fall back with cough and more toxins.
- Fever with a rash.

At the hospital, if you find a patient within 48 hours of the beginning of symptoms, a doctor can prescribe antivirals like adamantanes, such as amantadine and rimantadine (Flumadine), as well as flu inhibitors, like neuraminidase inhibitors, such as oseltamivir (Tamiflu) or zanamivir (Relenza) or peramivir and laninamivir (Inavir). The CDC advises that high-risk flu-like patients seek timely influenza anti-viral medicines without asking for test results to validate the flu.

Prevention

While daily hand washing and good hygiene techniques are effective to avoid influenza, the best path is to get the influenza vaccine each year. Researchers determine, each year, which influenza virus strain will be most involved and which vaccines should be developed to avoid infection.

The CDC suggests a regular flu vaccination for six months and older for all residents. "For seasonal flu, anyone younger, older, and immunocompromised, it is more probable to get flu; so if one in this category can not get vaccinated, it is necessary for others who have near connections with or care about them to get vaccinated in order to minimize risk," said Donelan.

So why do certain people always get influenza after a flu shot? The influenza vaccine helps defend against the most dangerous viruses in the given year. However, a type of virus may be transmitted, which is significantly distinct from that used in the seasonal vaccination.

Studies have also demonstrated that as pressures in the vaccine suit up with those in culture; vaccinated people are 60% less prone to get flu than those that are not vaccinated by the CDC.

And a 2013 report showed that screened people are less prone to have fewer symptoms.

Flu diagnosis

A doctor would usually inquire about their symptoms and perform a physical test if a person wants medical treatment for flu symptoms. A practitioner may even take a throat swab for examination.

The diagnostic test for fast influenza will yield result in 10-15 minutes, but may not be correct. More specific experiments will take longer to yield results.

Flu or a cold?

People sometimes confuse influenza for poor weather because certain signs are identical.

Cold and flu contain both:

- a runny or blocked nose
- a sore throat
- a cough
- chest discomfort
- fatigue

However, there are some differences:

- A cold does not involve a fever, while the flu usually does.
- The signs of a cold begin to occur slowly, although flu symptoms may grow rapidly.
- Cold symptoms are typically less severe than those of flu.
- A person can tend to feel exhausted for many weeks after getting influenza.

- Flu is most prone to trigger infections and life risks.

Flu or food poisoning?

Many kinds of viruses exist, and some may affect the digestive system. It's often referred to as "stomach hold," but varies from pneumonia, which is a respiratory illness.

The norovirus, which reaches the body by infected food or fluids, is the most common source of stomach flu. Nausea, vomiting, and diarrhea are signs. Similar signs are triggered by food poisoning.

Flu or pneumonia?

Pneumonia can be infectious or bacterial. Symptoms can sound like flu, but a person can feel intense, burning chest pain, particularly while he is breathing hard and coughing.

Slowly or unexpectedly, bacterial pneumonia may start. Symptoms can be:

- a very high temperature
- sweating
- rapid breathing and pulse rate
- blue nailbeds due to a lack of oxygen

Viral pneumonia signs are close to flu symptoms. They include:

- fever

- dry cough

- headache

- aches and weakness

By comparison to measles, though, pneumonia signs typically grow slowly. Someone with high temperature and trouble breathing should see a doctor right away.

Contagiousness

The flu virus transmits liquid droplets. A person will transfer the virus to anyone up to 6 feet away if he coughs, sneezes, talks, or breathes.

A safe individual will transmit the virus until they have symptoms themselves one day. In other terms, you will pass on the flu until you realize it. After signs arise, the infected individual may continue to spread the virus for up to 5-7 days.

Persons with a compromised immune system, older adults, and small children will transmit the virus faster than that. In the first 3–4 days after signs start, flu becomes most infectious.

Transmission

An individual may develop influenza symptoms if droplets containing the virus fall into their mouth, nose, or lungs from someone else's air.

This transmission can occur if:

- Someone without the virus is near a person with flu.

- A person who is virus-free approaches an item handled by a virus individual and then covers his lips, nose, or eyes.

- Evidence indicates that the flu virus can be transmitted only by coughing. Read more here. Know more here.

Incubation period

The duration of incubation of the disease is the time it takes for a person to be infected before the signs begin.

It's usually two days with flu, although it can range from 1 to 4 days. Even before symptoms occur, a human may spread the virus.

Flu when pregnant

Flu may be more severe during pregnancy because the activity of the immune system is impaired by pregnancy. If a woman is pregnant and has influenza, she may have to spend time in the hospital.

Complications linked to breastfeeding involve an increased chance of:

- preterm birth
- low birth weight
- stillbirth

In newborns, flu can be lethal. The mother's dangers include an elevated likelihood of problems such as bronchitis, ear, and blood infections.

How long is it going to last?

Flu signs spontaneously begin, typically about two days after infection. Within around one week, most signs resolve, but cough will continue for up to 2 weeks.

In certain instances, up to one week, after their symptoms are gone, an individual can still be infectious. Complications may take longer to overcome as they arise. Many of the most severe forms of injuries may have a long-term safety impact, such as kidney failure.

Many may experience post-viral tiredness for one week or two after the major effects. You may have a persistent feeling of tiredness and unhappiness.

Timeline

Typically, flu may progress as follows:

- The virus typically infects a human through the mouth or nose.
- We can be able to spread the virus to others after one day.
- Symptoms appear 1–2 days after infection.

- The probability of virus infection is the greatest three or four days after signs begin.

- After four days, the fever and muscle aches improve.

- After one week, most symptoms disappear.

- The possibility of infection spread declines five to seven days after signs.

- The cough and tiredness may remain for a further week.

Flu shot

The easiest approach to combat influenza is to get an influenza vaccine every year.

Two forms of vaccine exist:

The flu shot: A healthcare provider normally gives the flu shot in the neck using an injection. It's ideal for individuals older than six months, and for both able and seriously disabled individuals.

Vaccine for nasal spray flu: The flu vaccine for nasal sprays includes life-long, weakened flu viruses that do not trigger the disease.

According to the CDC, a flu shot may include multiple influenza virus vaccines.

Sources are:

- influenza A (H1N1) virus

- influenza (H3N2) virus
- one or two influenza B viruses

Viruses, though, evolve and alter with time, and scientists need to modify the vaccine material each year. International monitoring results allow experts to determine which forms will occur in a given flu season. Security begins roughly two weeks after the vaccine is obtained.

Vaccinations for seasonal flu will begin in September or until the vaccine is available. These start through the influenza season, in January and beyond.

Flu shot side effects

The CDC states that the influenza vaccine has a clear safety record and can not induce influenza. Following a vaccination, an individual can encounter the following adverse effects, although they should typically become mild within a few days.

- pain, redness, and swelling at the injection site
- headache
- fever
- nausea
- muscle aches

Approximately 1-2 people in 1 million can develop Guillain-Barr Syndrome (GBS). Individuals may still acquire GBS during influenza, though, and their chance is greater than that of the vaccine. For the nasal spray form of the vaccine, the chance of GBS will be smaller. When anyone has hives, swelling, and breathing problems following vaccination, they should receive prompt medical treatment because this is a symptom of an allergic reaction. A serious response is termed life-threatening anaphylaxis.

Flu shot pregnancy

Throughout breastfeeding, it is healthy to get the flu shot, and physicians suggest it. It takes approximately two weeks to cover. The shot often travels through the fetus, which defends them from the flu. Newborns never get a flu vaccine, but they may be unhealthy with influenza. Both mother and her unborn child will benefit from the vaccine.

Flu shot effectiveness

The flu shot can not offer 100% defense from grip since scientists can not correctly determine what forms of grip would occur over a season. The 2018–2019 CDC estimates indicate that the effectiveness of influenza A or B was about 47 percent.

Many variables will lead annually to the efficacy of the influenza shot. The age and fitness of the vaccine recipient and how closely the vaccination suits the predominant viruses should be used.

Flu shot for seniors

The CDC advises that individuals aged 65 years and over receive a flu shot. When individuals grow older, problems are more prone to occur because they have control.

Elders can require a higher dosage of vaccination because they are less likely to fight the flu virus in their immune systems. The vaccination is not entirely safe; however, it reduces the incidence of flu and the extent of complications.

A report in 2017 analyzed evidence for older patients in a hospital with influenza during the 2013-2014 flu season in the U.S. There were fewer deaths, fewer injuries, and fewer days spent in an intensive care unit for people who got the vaccine.

People aged 65 or older should question their physicians at the beginning of every flu season regarding the vaccine. The doctor should prescribe a specific vaccine.

Flu shot cost

The cost of an influenza shot in the private sector, depending on the form, is about $15–$24. And to figure out their protection, citizens will need to test their insurance plans. For starters, section B of Medicare pays for every flu season with one flu shot.

When to see a doctor

A doctor only needs to know that a person has the flu if:

- they are already frail or have an existing health condition
- they have a weakened immune system
- they are infants or aged 65 years or over
- their temperature remains high after 4–5 days
- symptoms worsen or are severe
- they become short of breath, develop chest pain or both

However, if you have questions about the effects, refer to the doctor for more guidance.

ORIGIN OF INFLUENZA

1. The Etymology of "Influenza"

The term influenza comes from the medieval Italian term for "influence" (influenza) and refers to the causes of the disease. *The English Dictionary of Oxford* notes that the origin or "influence" of the disease was originally deemed astrological, but the reason shifted with time to the "influence of the wind" (influenza del Freddo). The word "influenza" was originally found in the University of Edinburgh but was not widely used in Britain until the pandemic of 1782.

2. The First Pandemic (1580)

Scholars also discovered records about what seems to be at least 1173 C.E. outbreak flu, but the first influenza pandemic reported happened in 1580. Throughout the summer months, the pandemic started throughout Asia and quickly spread to Africa and then Europe via trade lines between Asia Minor to North Africa. Then the pandemic spread across Europe and the Atlantic to America during the next six months. For the time being, death rates remained staggeringly high. Academics claim that 9,000 fatalities happened only in Constantinople. Some accounts suggest that the entire populace of many Spanish towns were virtually eradicated.

3. Influenza in the 18th and 19th Centuries

More modern historical reports (since 1700) indicate a number of clear epidemics and pandemics of influenza that we are almost aware of. In spring 1729, an epidemic of influenza started in Russia and spread across Europe and finally across the globe in a three-year pandemic over the span of six months in western Europe. Another big pandemic broke out in China in the fall of 1781, until it traveled to Russia, and eventually to Europe during an eight-month pandemic. According to estimates, 30,000 citizens became sick each day in St. Petersburg at the height of the pandemic, and 2/3 of the city of Rome and 3/4 of those in Munich succumbed to the disease. Throughout the 19th century, Influenza began its pandemic outbreak in 1800-1802, 1830-33, 1847-1848, 1857-1858, and 1880-1890.

4. False Findings: An Etiological Error

When upwards of half of all German townspeople developed at least a mild influenza outbreak, during the pandemic of 1880-1890, a German surgeon called Richard Pfeiffer began taking reports from his patients with nasal discharge. In 1892, he cultivated a bacterium from those samples, which he named Bacillus influenza (or Pfeiffer's bacillus, more often). This bacterium, which we now know as Haemophilus influenza, was believed by Pfeiffer to be the cause of the pandemic influenza.

In fact, Haemophilus influenza was not responsible for viral influenza. But the bacteria caused opportunistic local infections only in a previously impaired immune system, such as a patient with influenza. Because anthrax, cholera, and tuberculosis bacteria had recently been identified, and since there was a shortage of an appropriate microscope to detect slightly smaller viruses, very few of his colleagues questioned the observations of Pfeiffer, and his bacterial etiology became recognized as the source of the pandemic influenza in the future.

5. The 1918-1919 Pandemic: A History by the Numbers

The XXth century witnessed the two most significant case studies in the world of infectious diseases: the influenza pandemic of 1918-1919 and the worldwide epidemic with HIV / AIDS at the end of the 20th century. In the implacable 1918-1919 pandemic, influenza made its historical impact. This struck the end of the First World War, which from 1914-1918 claimed the lives of 10 million soldiers. A new study indicates that influenza has claimed the lives of more than 30 million citizens globally — and far less than the conflict itself. During the pandemic, more people died of influenza in one year than the entire Black Death period (1347-1351), which eradicated about 30-60% of the whole of Europe. In England alone, over 225,000 people suffered from influenza between 1918 and 1919.

6. Why "Spanish Flu"?

We also learn about the 1918-1919 influenza pandemic called "The Spanish flu." The first influenza cases arose far from neutral Spain at Fort Riley Military Base in Kansas, though. Unit cook Albert Gitchell registered sick with a fever of 40°C at Fort Riley's Camp

Funston on 4 March 1918. In days, 522 people registered sick, and 1,100 soldiers were admitted to the influenza hospital by the end of the month. Of these, 237 acquired pneumonia, and 38 died (approximately 20 percent). Therefore, if the pandemic started in California, then was the "Spanish Flu" alluded to? Historians are now arguing this misnomer, although the most plausible reason is that Spain was dying early and murdered 8 million citizens in May 1918 with a significant amount of casualties.

7. 1918-1919 as a Public Health Crisis

The pandemic of 1918–1919 soon covered the world, with much of society witnessing the symptoms of flu via trade roads and rail lines. Through its dawn and demobilization, the Great War accelerated the fast dissemination of the pandemic. Outbreaks also spread across the South Pacific, North America, Europe, Asia, Africa, and Brazil. A lack of physicians, particularly in the civil sector, was a popular occurrence, as many were lost to military service.

At the end of August 1918, the pandemic viral transformation happened in Brest, France (22 August), Freetown, Sierra Leone (24 August), and Boston, Massachusetts (27 August). Death ended at the end of autumn 1918. Those fortunate enough to avoid contamination needed to comply with public health laws to stop the disease spread: government offices issued gauze masks to be used in public; stores were forbidden to conduct sales; funerals were restricted to 15 minutes. Some cities needed a signed certificate to join, and without them, railways would not welcome passengers. Those who disregarded flu laws had to face substantial fines.

8. Finding the Viral Cause

In the pandemic of 1918-1919, scientists believed that the cause was the latest strain of Pfeiffer bacillus, but only a limited number of patient reports displayed samples of bacillus. Following the pandemic, scientists revived the thesis on influenza etiology. In 1931, an American virologist, Richard Shope, made a major discovery: the influenza A virus mutation in pigs. Patrick Laidlaw was appointed to the United Kingdom Scientific Study Council two years later. The Shope and Laidlaw laboratories described the H1N1 influenza A virus, which eventually triggered the 1918-1919 pandemic, together in 1935-1936.

9. The Quest for a Vaccine

In 1919, physicians attempted to vaccinate influenza patients by creating a bacillus vaccine for Pfeiffer, but this turned out to be completely unsuccessful for the wrong reason. In view of the detection of viral influenza by Shope and Laidlaw, scientists began focusing on a modern influenza vaccine almost instantly. Ernest Goodpasture, a pathology professor at the University of Vanderbilt, started breeding the virus in hen eggs in 1931. This research became important to the creation of the first modern flu vaccines. Initially developed by the U.S. forces during the Second World War, influenza vaccinations were only introduced in general in the 1950s. Although egg culture technology is still in use, the FDA authorized a virus growth in cell cultures as of 2012.

10. Swine Flu, or Why You Should Get a Flu Shot

A new H1N1 strain appeared in Mexico in Spring 2009 and spread quickly across the globe. Millions of patients were infected, but death levels stayed smaller than just seasonal influenza. However, this seems to be a different form of the same virus that triggered the big 1918-1919 pandemic that destroyed so many millions of citizens. Fortunately, scientists were able to grow the viral strain very rapidly. As a consequence, the regular flu shot even defends against the H1N1 flu virus. When physicians are worried about a fresh pandemic, make sure that you have a flu shot.

INFLUENZA PANDEMICS IN HISTORY

Many patients with influenza have been feeling sick for a couple of days and eventually heal. In some cases, flu can lead to pneumonia, other complications, and even death.

People's defense from viruses relies on the virus being transmitted to them previously, through contamination or by viral vaccination. The immune system "remembers" the infection in any situation and generates infection-specific antibodies that neutralize the virus as it eventually reaches the body. However, influenza viruses can rapidly mutate or alter. Influenza viruses mutate several years to create a new type. This cycle is referred to as antigenic drift. Many subjected to a similar strain of the virus would presumably have pre-existing immunity in the form of antibodies, and the disease that occurs would be moderate.

Occasionally, a significant shift in a virus creates such a strain that people had little to no natural tolerance before. This phase is known as antigenic shift and may contribute to a specific, severe disease.

An influenza epidemic happens after an antigenic change produces a new subtype or strain of the influenza virus, which spreads worldwide. In the 20th century, three pandemics existed, all of them triggered by antigenic influenza A strains. A 2009 pandemic that was less lethal than the diseases of the 20th century was the product of a rare mix of genetic shifts. The 1918-19 pandemic is the case to which the death count in any subsequent pandemics is unparalleled.

Spanish Influenza, 1918-19

No other outbreak took as many lives as the 1918-1919 Spanish influenza epidemic. Worldwide, approximately 40 million citizens died, when this virulent disease reached city by city (almost 70 million deaths is estimated). There are loads of stories of individuals suffering within hours of first falling sick. The mortality risk was greatest in individuals under the age of 50 who were especially susceptible to severe influenza disease for unexplained reasons.

In early spring 1918, the first outbreaks of influenza arose in Kansas. Later in the spring, officials reported more reports from Europe, although this flu did not appear to be more severe than usual. In late summer, though, the virus was more lethal. Arms of diseases soon moved across towns, countries, and continents, crippling clinics, and medical staff. In the autumn of 1918, the term Spanish flu originated from the devastating effects of the flu in Spain.

There was no medication nor an appropriate antidote for influenza in 1918. In reality, most scientists assumed that instead of a virus, it was a bacterium induced influenza. While several other diseases have had vaccinations, several ineffective and potentially harmful influenza vaccines have been planned, a successful influenza vaccine has been produced for decades. There were no antibiotics for the management of virulent bacterial infections that arose as a consequence of influenza.

The last Spanish influenza was seen in the late spring of 1919. The virus migrated through the 1920s into relative harmlessness and proceeded to spread for several decades. Since then, scientists have been willing to identify the 1918-19 pandemic virus as H1N1 influenza.

Asian Influenza, 1957-58

Annually after the 1918 pandemic, influenza persisted, but there were no fresh and virulent influenza forms until early 1957. Signs started to surface in February of that year of a severe outbreak of flu entering China.

The Walter Reed Army Medical Center microbiologist, Maurice Hilleman, found press stories on influenza in Asia. The number of reports prompted him to conclude that a different strain of influenza arose and caused a pandemic.

Hilleman and his colleagues collected an American serviceman report of the infection. They soon figured out that most citizens lacked antibody defense against the recent H2N2 type influenza virus. Only some older people who survived the 1889-1890 flu pandemic displayed an antibody response to the new virus.

Hilleman started to create a vaccine by giving producers virus samples and advising them to establish a vaccine within four months.

In October 1957, when around 7 million citizens were vaccinated, the U.S. outbreak hit the peak. About 2 million people globally perished from Asian flu from 1957 to 1958, including about 70,000 fatalities in the United States.

Hong Kong Flu, 1968-69

Like the pandemic just ten years ago, the first symptoms of a modern form of influenza A appeared in Asia. In September 1968, the virus (H3N2) entered the US and emerged in the winter months. A vaccine was developed but was not manufactured early enough to provide sufficient safety. Around 34,000 people perished during this pandemic in the United States. Some scientists suggest the correlations with Asian flu in 1957-58 may have led to shielding citizens from more severe diseases. (Like the Asian flu, the N2 part of Hong Kong flu)

Avian Flu Threat, 1997-Present

The next big danger of influenza originated from Asia, where birds were contaminated by avian influenza (H5N1) and later transmitted to humans. Many individuals got sick and died of the flu.

The outbreaks in 2003-2004 were especially serious, as tens of millions of poultry and waterfowl died of flu. The virus did not spread from person to person, however, but only among birds and then among people. The lack of human-to-human infections extended to a minimal degree. The hazard decreased after the widespread loss of poultry flocks. However, the possibility of bird flu shows that another deadly outbreak could occur, which might spread to humans and spark a pandemic.

Novel H1N1, 2009

The new influenza pandemic erupted in Mexico in mid-March 2009. The flu first appeared especially alarming because mortality levels were extraordinarily large in Mexico. Throughout California and Texas, outbreaks soon arose, and the epidemic began to propagate. Scientists described the virus as H1N1 influenza, possibly of pig origin.

The World Health Organisation issued global updates on the evolving crisis, and pandemic influenza preparations started to be introduced at regional, state, and local levels. While the disease progressed quickly at an initial height at the beginning of May in the United States, the resulting disease did not appear to be as serious as early Mexican reports suggested. The disease has still taken a heavier toll on children and young adults than typical seasonal flu. In total, 90 percent of seasonal flu-related deaths occur in persons over the age of 65, while 87 percent of H1N1 deaths occur in persons under the age of 65. A potential reason for this is because many individuals born before 1950, possibly because virus forms identified with the H1N1 pandemic of 1918 were already prevalent earlier in the 20th century, tended to have preexisting tolerance to the virus.

After scientists established the virus, a major undertaking to develop a vaccine for the latest strain H1N1 began. Throughout the development cycle, the virus displayed a sluggish growth that relies on the cultivation of the virus in chicken eggs. In the United States, the bulk of doses arrived in late October during the second influenza season. Scientists had previously estimated that by mid-October 160 million doses of the vaccine would be eligible. But just 30 million doses were distributed at the point.

Around April 2009 and February 13, 2010, CDC reported that around 42 million and 86 million instances of 2009 H1N1 existed in the United States. During this time, between 188,000 and 389,000 hospitalizations were performed, as were 8,520-17,620 deaths.

Was H1N1 the result of antigenic change or antigenic drift in 2009? There was no new H- or N-subtype that would suggest an antigenic change. Nevertheless, the virus obviously does not adhere to the concept of antigenic drift. "The appearance of the H1N1 virus in 2009 is an extraordinary phenomenon in contemporary virology. The 2009 H1N1 virus does not adhere to the standard concept of a viral subtype, as certain patients do not have prior infections. H1N1 has been in continuous circulation since 1977, and most people born before 1956 undergo H1N1 infection in the pre-H2N2 period. The 2009 H1N1 virus also does not meet the standard drift concept because it has no clear genetic association with the recent distribution of human H1N1 viruses." (Sullivan SJ, Jacobson RM, Dowdle WR, Poland GA. 2009 H1N1 Influenza).

In 2005, the World Health Organisation established updated pandemic recommendations to reconsider and update the preparations for pandemic preparedness in national and local authorities. The preparations were created after the epidemic of bird flu in the late 1990s. The 2009 H1N1 pandemic was stable. Governments have the potential to develop innovative strategies to respond to pandemic disease.

As groups research the 2009 pandemic response, several refer to the need for accelerated influenza vaccine production and delivery. Advanced techniques and strategies for increasing the supply of vaccinations are being studied by business and public health authorities. As in the EU and Canada, for example, US companies might consider using an adjuvant for the influenza vaccine, which will enable them to use smaller doses of antigen for any dose. In fact, modern antigen collection techniques may be used to stop the sluggish method of developing vaccines in eggs.

There is an apparent need for continued commitment to pandemic influenza preparations. As a Unified Nation, "If the pandemic influenza virus originated with a comparable virulence to the 1918 strain now, it is projected that in the lack of action, 1,9 million Americans could be infected and almost 10 million hospitalized." (Pandemic Influenza Program of the US Department of Health and Human Services).

SPANISH FLU

The most deadly pandemic in history, the Spanish flu pandemic of 1918, has infected approximately 500 million people worldwide – about a third of the planet's population – killing an estimated 20 million to 50 million people, including some 675,000 Americans. Throughout Germany, the United States, and areas of Asia, grip throughout 1918 was first recorded until it quickly expanded across the globe. At the moment, no appropriate medications or treatments are available to combat the killer flu virus. Citizens have been told to carry gloves, classrooms, theaters, and businesses, and bodies have been locked up in fortuitous morgues until the epidemic begins its lethal global march.

What Is the Flu?

Flu is an infection that affects the respiratory system. The flu virus is extremely contagious: When a sick person dances, sneezes, or speaks, coughing droplets are produced and spread into the air and can then be inhaled by anyone in the area.

In fact, a person who absorbs the virus and covers his or her lips, eyes, or nose may get contaminated.

During the 1918 influenza pandemic, the Health Commissioner in New York City sought to stop the outbreak in flu by ordering corporations to open and shut phased shifts in order to prevent overcrowding in subways.

Grippe outbreaks arise each year and differ according to the form of the virus that spreads. (Flu viruses will mutate quickly.)

Flu Season

Across the USA, "flu season" typically takes place from late fall to spring. In the average year, more than 200 000 Americans have been treated with flu-related complications, and over the last three decades, according to the Centers for Disease Control and Prevention, about 3,000 to 49,000 US flu-related deaths were registered last year.

Youths aged 65 and younger are at greater risk of flu-related infections, including cough, ear, sinus and bronchitis, and those with other medical conditions such as asthma, diabetes, or heart failure.

A flu pandemic, such as that of 1918, happens when a highly virulent new form of influenza that loses or has no tolerance is discovered and is rapidly transmitted around the globe.

Spanish Flu Symptoms

Throughout the spring, the first outbreak of the 1918 pandemic took place and was generally moderate. The patients with such common influenza symptoms as chills, fever, and tiredness, typically healed after a few days and registered low deaths.

In the fall of the same year, though, a second extremely infectious outbreak of influenza emerged with a vengeance. Victims died in hours or days after signs, their skin turned gray, and their lungs were filled with fluid, which caused them to suffocate. In just one year, 1918, America's average life expectancy fell by a dozen years.

What Caused the Spanish Flu?

This remains unclear precisely where the specific influenza virus that started this pandemic came from, although it was first detected in Germany, America and parts of Asia in 1918, until it spread to almost every other region of the planet over a matter of months.

While influenza in 1918 has not been limited to one area, it has been recognized across the world as Spanish flu, because Spain has been seriously impacted by the disease and not prone to wartime news outages which have impacted many European countries. (Alfonso XIII, the king of Spain, also reportedly caught influenza.) Another peculiar feature of the 1918 influenza was that it affected several previously stable young men — a category that was usually immune to certain contagious diseases— including many World War I soldiers.

Yes, more U.S. troops suffered from pneumonia in 1918 than they were killed in the fighting. Forty percent in the United States Navy became struck by fever, although 36% of the Army was sick, and soldiers in cramped vessels and railways across the globe helped spread the deadly epidemic.

Although the death rate of Spanish influenza is mostly reported at 20 to 50 million globally, some figures are 100 million – around 3 percent of the world's population. The precise figures are not established because of a shortage of medical information in certain countries.

What is clear, though, is that few areas were immune to 1918 influenza — in America, citizens from big towns to rural Alaskan communities endured as a result. Also, President Woodrow Wilson was stated to have grasped during the talks of the Versailles Treaty, ending World War I, in early 1919.

Why Was The Spanish Flu Called The Spanish Flu?

The Spanish flu did not originate from Mexico, but it was featured in the press. Throughout the First World War, Spain was a neutral nation with international media reporting the war from the outset and published in Madrid for the first time in late May 1918. Meanwhile, the Allied countries and the Central Powers had war censors that covered up reports of flu to preserve strong moral values. Although Spanish news outlets were the only ones that mentioned flu, many assumed that it emerged from there (the Spanish claimed that the virus came from France and named it a 'French flu').

Where Did The Spanish Flu Come From?

Scientists also do not know with certainty where the Spanish flu emerged, while hypotheses point to France, China, Great Britain, or the US, where the first recorded case was registered in Fort Riley, Kansas, on March 11, 1918.

Some suspect that untreated soldiers distributed the disease around the country to other military camps and took it abroad. Throughout March 1918, 84,000 U.S. soldiers entered the Atlantic, and 118,000 more arrived the following month.

Fighting the Spanish Flu

When the 1918 grip hit, physicians and scientists were unsure about what caused it or how it was treated. Contrary to the current situation, there were no effective vaccines or antivirals, medicines that treat influenza. Throughout America, the first approved flu vaccine was developed in the '40s. Over the following decade, suppliers of vaccinations regularly developed vaccinations that could better monitor and deter potential pandemics. This was complicated by the fact that areas of America had been left with a lack of doctors and other healthcare professionals in World War I. And many of the available U.S. medical staff came down with flu.

In fact, clinics became so overwhelmed with grip patients in certain places that schools, private homes, and other facilities turned into change clinics.

Officials in certain cities enforced quarantines, required the residents, including schools, churches, and theatres, to wear masks and shut public spaces. They were told to quit raising their hands to sit inside, so the libraries started lending books.

Boy Scouts in New York City, according to the NYT, confronted men they noticed smoking on the ground and issued them cards reading, "You break the sanitary code" during the pandemic.

What advice were people given?

Doctors forgot what their patients would recommend; several doctors advised people to avoid busy areas or literally some. Many treatments also involved spice feeding, wine drinking, or even meat consumption from Oxo (beef broth). Physicians advised patients to keep their ears and nose completely hidden. At one point, the use of medication was suspected of triggering the pandemic, though it may have protected the sick population.

On 28 June 1918, a public notice appeared in the British papers that advised people about the symptoms of influenza; however, this was actually a Formamints advertisement, a tablet manufactured and sold by a vitamin company. Just when people aged, there was wealth to be gained from false remedies. Minting was proclaimed to be the "only way of preventing contagious diseases," so everyone, including babies, would suck four to five of such pills a day before they felt stronger.

Specific guidance was given to Americans about how to prevent infection. They were told not to shake hands, sit indoors, do not contact library books, and wear masks. Schools and theaters closed, and the New York Department of Health strictly enforced the update to the Sanitary Code, which, according to an article reported in the newspaper Public Health Records, made street spitting unlawful.

The Spanish Flu

World War I contributed to a lack of physicians in some regions, with many of the patients sick. Schools and other facilities were converted into renovation clinics, and in some instances, medical students were needed to substitute physicians.

How many civilians were killed?

By the spring of 1919, the number of Spanish influenza deaths declined. Countries were left ravaged because medical practitioners were powerless to avoid the transmission of the disease after the epidemic. The pandemic repeated 500 years ago as the Black Death created panic all over the world.

How do you equate this with seasonal influenza?

Spanish flu is still the deadliest influenza pandemic to date, killing about 1% to 3% of the world's population.

The last flu pandemic emerged in 2009-2010, following the emergence of a new H1N1 influenza virus. The disease has been dubbed the "swine grasp" because the virus causing this disease is identical to the one present in pigs.

Swine flu triggered respiratory infections, which, according to the Centers for Disease Prevention and Control, killed an estimated 151,700-575,400 people worldwide in the first year. It was only 0.001 percent or 0.007 percent of the world's population, and the pandemic was slightly less severe than the Spanish influenza pandemic of 1918. About 80 percent of swine flu fatalities were rare among people younger than 65. Typically, 70-90 percent of seasonal influenza deaths occur in people older than 65.

An annual influenza vaccine is now included in the influenza strain that causes swine flu. Every year people often suffer from flu, but on average, the figures are significantly smaller than those for swine flu or Spanish influenza pandemics. According to the World Health Organization, global epidemics of seasonal flu result in around 3 to 5 million serious cases and between 290,000 to 650,000 fatalities.

Aspirin Poisoning and the Flu

Since there was no treatment for flu, a lot of physicians recommended medicines that they thought would reduce complications, including the introduction of aspirin by the Bayer family in 1899, which had ended in 1917, which implies that after the Spanish flu outbreak, new businesses manufactured the product.

Until the increase in deaths triggered by Spanish flu in 1918, the United States Surgeon General, Navy, and the American Medical Association Report also advised that aspirin be used. Health specialists also recommended patients to take a dosage of up to 30 grams a day, which is considered to be harmful. The signs of aspirin toxicity include either hyperventilation and pulmonary edema or an excess of fluid in the lung, and it is widely suspected that much of the deaths in October were probably triggered or hastened by aspirin toxicity.

The Flu Takes Heavy Toll on Society

Grippe took a huge toll on men, wiping out whole households, leaving countless widows and orphans behind. Funeral spaces were crowded, and corpses were rounded up. For their own family members, often, citizens had to dig graves.

Grippe was often detrimental to the market. Businesses in the United States needed to close down because too many workers became injured. Based on affected staff, essential utilities such as postal delivery and garbage collection were hampered.

There were not enough agricultural staff in certain areas to grow crops. Also, state and municipal health services remained inaccessible to corporations, which hampered attempts to chronicle the outbreak of grip in 1918 and give responses to the public.

How U.S. Cities Tried to Stop The 1918 Flu Pandemic

Throughout the summer of the year 1918, a catastrophic second outbreak of Spanish Flu struck the U.S. when re-entered veterans afflicted with the disease transmitted it to the general public, especially throughout heavily populated towns. The local mayors and health officers devised strategies to secure their residents' safety without vaccination or approved treatment programs. Despite the motivation to remain loyal during the war and filtered media to minimize the transmission of the epidemic, many made disastrous decisions.

The response from Philadelphia was too little, too late. Dr. Wilmer Krusen, the city's head of public safety and charity, claimed that the deaths that would escalate were not caused by "Spanish flu," but rather common flu. Thus, the city proceeded on 18 September with a Liberty Loan parade witnessed by thousands of Philadelphians, spreading the epidemic like wildfires. More than 1,000 Philadelphians perished in just ten days, leaving 200,000 more hospitalized. Only then did the town shutter the theaters and saloons. By March 1919, more than 15,000 Philadelphia residents had lost their lives.

St. Louis, Missouri, was different: colleges and museums were closed down, and public hearings were prohibited. The overall mortality rate in Saint Louis, however, was just one-eighth of the death rate in Philadelphia at the pandemic period.

The residents of San Francisco were fined $5 – a big number in those days – because they were found without masks in public and charged with disrupting order.

Spanish Flu Pandemic Ends

By the summer of 1919, the influenza pandemic began, when sick people perished or gained immunity.

In 2008, almost 90 years later, researchers announced that they had found out what made the 1918 flu so deadly: a group of three genes allowed the virus to weaken the bronchial tubes and lungs of the victim and to clear the way for bacterial pneumonia.

The Spanish Flu

Several other influenza pandemics, but none as severe, have arisen since 1918. Between 1957 and 1958, an influenza pandemic killed about 2 million people around the world, including about 70,000 in the United States, and between 1968 and 1969, a pandemic killed around 1 million people and about 34,000 Americans.

About 12,000 people were infected during the 2009-2010 H1N1 (or "swine flu") pandemic. The latest 2020 coronavirus pandemic occurs around the globe with countries rushing to cure COVID 19 and residents sheltering in an effort to prevent transmitting the disease, which is particularly dangerous as many carriers remain asymptomatic for days prior to their diagnosis.

Each of the current pandemics brings fresh focus and concern in Spanish flu, or "forgotten pandemic," so-called because its outbreak was overshadowed by the deadliness of WWI.

HISTORY OF 1918 SPANISH FLU

The 1918-1919 influenza pandemic killed more people than any other disease outbreak in existence in absolute numbers. A current estimate shows 21 million fatalities, a statistic that remains in the media today, which highlights the true number. This statistic has since been updated many times by epidemiologists and scientists. All of the updates have been upward. Frank Macfarlane Burnet, who received his Nobel Prize in Immunology but spent the better part of his life researching flu, claimed that the death toll was potentially 50 million and perhaps 100 million. An epidemiological study in 2002 reports that fatalities vary from 50 million to 100 million.

Throughout 1918, the world's population was only 28% of the population today. An equivalent toll today would be between 175 and 350 million for the nation. By comparison, around 24 million people have been killed by AIDS, and an estimated 40 million people have been infected with the virus.

A message from a specialist in one U.S. military camp for a colleague puts a more human face on those numbers: These men begin with what would seem to be an ordinary LaGrippe or Influenza attack and if brought into the hospital, quickly develop the most dangerous type of pneumonia ever seen ... and a few hours later you can start looking at Cyanosis stretching from their ears and spreading across their face until it is hard. It's only a few hours until death comes... It's bad. You may bear to see one, two or 20 men die, but to see these little devils dropping like flies... We have reported nearly 100 deaths a day... Pneumonia causes mortality in any situation... We lost an incredible amount of nurses and physicians. Special trains are expected to hold the dead. There were no coffins for many days, and the corpses stacked up against something terrible... It hit every vision they'd ever had during a war in France. An extra-large barracks was cleared for the use of the morgue so that everyone might sit down and take care of the long lines of dead soldiers all suited up and lined in double rows ... Nice by ancient Friend, Heaven is with you before we see you again.

This letter represented a traditional encounter in the cantonments of the American Army. The background of everyday life was not any easier.

It is important to investigate developments in 1918 in readiness for another pandemic for observations, alerts, and places for further study.

The 1918 pandemic was hardly the first or only fatal influenza pandemic. In literature, there have been pandemics of pneumonia, some of which may have rivaled the death of 1918. A partial list of particularly violent influenza outbreaks was one in 1510 when a pandemic suspected to have been from Africa "at once struck and raged all over Europe without losing a family and with a few men." In 1580, an additional pandemic started in Asia and then traveled to Africa, Europe, and even America (although it took six weeks to cross the ocean). This was so serious that "almost all the countries in Europe, of which only the twenties was safe from the epidemic," endured within six weeks, and several Spanish towns were "almost completely depopulated by the epidemic." In 1688, influenza hit England, Ireland, and Virginia; "men frowned as in plague" in all these areas. In 1693, a modified or new epidemic again infected Europe and America, and in 1699 Massachusetts. "Many households suffered from illness. None survived and in some communities, many died particularly in Cambridge, some oddly if uniquely, in certain cities, nearly all were sick, and it was a period of sickness. Throughout England, more citizens perished of flu throughout 1847 and 1848 than the devastating 1832 cholera outbreak. A huge and deadly worldwide pandemic occurred again in 1889 and 1890."

Yet 1918 seems particularly brutal. It started slowly, with a spring storm. Yes, it was so slight that some physicians asked if it was influenza. In separate journal papers, usually, some Italian doctors claimed that "the febrile fever currently commonly widespread in Italy [is] not influenza." In July 1918, the Lancet report concluded that the spring outbreak was not influenza, because the effects, while like influenza, were "quite brief and thus far free from relapse or complications."

A second pandemic outbreak spread across the globe within a few weeks of this report in Lancet. It even led researchers to suspect whether influenza was the epidemic, except this time because it was so virulent. Followed by the third outbreak in 1919, a significant epidemic also emerged in 1920. The virus from 1918, notably in their second wave, was not only virulent and deadly but also highly violent (victims of the first wave provided great tolerance to the second and third waves, giving convincing proof that both were triggered by the same virus). This developed a variety of signs never associated with the disease. After H5N1 first occurred in 1997, pathologists reported "not previously described with influenza" findings. In addition, researchers mentioned any changes in pathology seen with H5N1 and more in 1918.

Symptoms in 1918 were so rare that dengue, cholera, or typhoid was originally misdiagnosed. An author wrote, "Hemorrhaging from mucous membranes, particularly the nose, stomach, and intestine, was one of the more disturbing complications. Bleeding from the ears and petechial bleeding often happened in the head." A German investigator reported with great frequency "hemorrhages in different sections of the inside of the eye." An American pathologist noted: "Fifty sub-conjunctival hemorrhage cases have been reported. Twelve had a perfect hemorrhage, vivid red blood without any mucus admixture..." There was bowel hemorrhage in three instances. New York City's chief pathologist said, "Cases with extreme pain look and function like dengue ... nasal or bronchial hemorrhage ... brain or spinal paralysis ... mobility loss may be serious or moderate, chronic, or acute ... physical and mental distress. Intense, chronic prostration contributes to suicidal depression, despair, and insanity."

The influenza of 1918 also infected young people. South African cities accounted for 60% of deaths between 20 and 40 years. Throughout Chicago, the suicides of 20 to 40-year-olds are about five times those of 41 to 60-year-olds. Throughout the "registration area" of the US — the states and cities that held accurate statistics — the highest number of deaths happened in the population between 25 and 29 years old, the second largest of them in the period of 30 to 34 years old, and the third in the age category between 20 and 24 years old. Further, citizens died in both of these five-yellow categories than the cumulative fatalities of those over the age of 60 and the aggregate fatalities of 20-34 of those over the age of 50. If tainted, the single party would most definitely perish. The mortality rate ranged from 23 to 71 percent in 13 trials of adult pregnant people during the 1918 pandemic. Of the surviving pregnant women, 26% lost their baby. (As far back as 1557, influenza was linked with pregnancy and the deaths of pregnant women.) The mortality rate for the disease was high. The average number can not be collected or even accurately calculated since there are no reliable statistics on cumulative events. Case mortality always surpassed 5% at U.S. Army camps where relatively accurate figures are kept and, in some instances, reached 10%. Case mortality for white troops was 9.6 percent in the British Army in India, while for Indian troops, it was 21.9 percent.

The infection killed infected people at much higher levels. In 16 days, 14% of the total people of the Fiji Islands disappeared. In Newfoundland and Greenland, at least one-third of the whole tribal community was destroyed.

Although probably the most troubling and perhaps important point now is that a large number —and a plurality of some subgroups

The Spanish Flu

of the population — died directly from the infection rather than from secondary bacterial pneumonia.

In 1918, pathologists became well acquainted with the lung state of patients of bacterial pneumonia after autopsy. And infectious pneumonia triggered by the influenza pandemic was so severe that the only lungs they had became casualties of poison gas.

So the army called them "atypical pneumonia." Now we'd term that atypical pneumonia the ARDS. The Pneumonia Board of the Army held that "about half" of all soldiers' lives were affected by this atypical pneumonia.

This can not be extrapolated to the general community explicitly. Army estimates, like overcrowded castles, are a special case both in terms of people and climate.

However, it's a sign that ARDS actually triggered about half the deaths of young people. ARDS mortality rates today vary from 40 and 60%, even with assistance in modern ICUs. In a pandemic, ICUs will be resolved easily, posing a significant obstacle for policymakers in public health.

Physicians have used all of their expertise, all they've learned, including the ancient art of bleeding patients, oxygen management, creation of modern vaccines and sera (mainly Hemophilusinfluenzae — a term originally called the etiological agent — and numerous pneumococci types). There was only one clinical intervention, which demonstrated little effectiveness by transfusing blood from the treated patients to fresh victims.

George Whipple, later Nobel Prize laureate, researched and considered a variety of vaccinations and drugs 'without treatment,' but he said from some vaccinations, "Static data indicates the possibility ... of any prophylactic value." Two other bacterial vaccines might have avoided specific secondary pneumonia.

In the meantime, any definition was used by the public at home. None showed any evidence of influence.

Some non-medical methods were effective. Complete separation, which removes a group from the outside environment, served as early as possible. Gunnison, Colorado, a railway village big enough to include a town, managed to separate itself. That's also what Fairbanks did in Alaska. American Samoa survived without a single occurrence, and 22 percent of the whole community perished a hundred miles south in Western Samoa.

More noteworthy – and even more significant – an Army analysis found that it was "unattainably enforced when and where" to separate both human victims and whole commands including contaminated troops, however "had nice ... when and where rigidly carried out" (Soper, undated draft report).

While isolation just slowed the virus, it was worth it. One of the epidemiological observations most significant in 1918 was the later in the second phase, the less probable it was to die and the milder the disease became.

This was possible because the virus entered a certain region late in the second wave and, more interestingly, was valid even inside that field. That is, towns affected later appeared to struggle less, so residents in that area later hurt fewer. Thus, the West Coast American towns infected later, had lower mortality rates than those on East Coast, and Australia had the lowest death rates in any developing nation, not affected by the second wave until 1919.

Again, interestingly, a person who got sick in one place for four days in an epidemic was more likely to develop viral pneumonia, which progressed to ARDS than a person who got sick in that place for four weeks. We were also prone to contract and suffer from secondary bacterial pneumonia.

The best data on this is from the United States. For the 20 main cantonments of the Army, nearly 20 percent of all influenza soldiers acquired pneumonia in the first five affected. Among all, 37.3% perished.

Across the last five centers, just 7.1% of influenza patients reported pneumonia, an average of 3 weeks back. Just 17.8% of the soldiers who contracted pneumonia were killed.

The same pattern extended inside the growing camp. The soldiers hit early died significantly more than the soldiers hit late in the same area.

The first towns — Boston, Baltimore, Pittsburgh, Philadelphia, Louisville, New York, New Orleans, and smaller towns — all operated in the same way. Across these same areas, though, the individuals infected by influenza during the outbreak did not get as sick and did not suffer at the same pace as those afflicted within the first two or three weeks.

The areas impacted by the outbreak typically saw lower mortality rates. In Connecticut, one of the most diligent epidemiological research was performed. The investigator stated that the similarity to the first epidemic in New London, when the disease was first imported to Connecticut, "is a consideration that seemed to affect the mortality rate..." The virus was more virulent or quickly spread as it first came into the state and then was usually attenuated.

The same trend spread around the nation and the planet. This wasn't a static prediction. The infection was never completely accurate. Nonetheless, areas reached later were less likely to fail.

One possible theory that may clarify why is that patient treatment has changed because community professionals have studied how to interact with this epidemic. But after analysis, this theory collapses. In a given area, medical treatment disintegrated throughout the epidemic. Doctors and nurses became overworked and ill, and patients, maybe most of them, got little treatment in the event of illness.

Also, in military bases, where contact could be required from physicians from bases to camps, there seemed to be no changes in medical treatment that could compensate for the differing mortality levels. A renowned scholar expressly searched for and found no proof of increased health or effective prevention strategies in military camps.

A second apparent causal theory is still disappointing that the most disadvantaged persons were first affected. To prove this theory valid, Americans on the east coast were more vulnerable than those on the west shore, and Americans and Western Europeans were more vulnerable than Australians.

Yet another possibility may be worth pursuing, albeit fully hypothetical. When you think back and glance at the history of the United States, it appears like civilians around the world experienced the most serious assaults in September and in early October. Many contaminated subsequently endured less in whatever region of the world they were.

During the height of the pandemic, the virus also continued to mutate exponentially, almost every time the human was shipped, so it was mutating into a less deadly shape.

We know that a lethal virus developed after a mild spring wave and a certain number of human passages. It could have been less virulent after additional passages. That would be especially helpful because the virus became latent as it exploded in September, just a couple of months before the deadly wave reached the human community.

This theory can indicate other study areas.

Social Disruption and Public Health Lessons

The disease was poorly treated in the United States, with the nternational and local authorities, and the public health agencies, providing a valuable case study.

The history is significant. Each government involved in the First World War had been attempting to regulate public opinion. In order to stop harming morality, also in the first non-lethal surge, the epidemic of countries fighting the war was not reported. (But Spain was not at war, and the newspapers reported it, and it was called Spanish flu).

There was little disparity in the United States. In 1917 Senator Hiram Johnson of California made a popular statement that "the first casualty of war is real." U.S. Congress enacted a statute that rendered it punishable by 20 years in jail to "talk, print, compose or publish some disloyal, political, scurrilous or offensive words against the United States 'congress." A Senator was arrested. Around the same period, the government launched a major campaign project.

An architect said, "Truth and lies are meaningless without fact. The power of a concept resides in its motivational nature. It doesn't matter whether it's real or not."

The mixture of strict discipline and loss of regard for reality had negative repercussions. Public leaders almost always concentrated on the shorter word and claimed half-truths or straight-out lies to prevent undermining morals and war efforts. The press embraced them, not opposed, who, while not legally controlled, cooperated entirely with the government's war machine.

Routinely, as influenza entered a city or community — one might watch it march any place— municipal authorities originally advised the people not to panic. They were stopped from getting affected by the illness by public health agencies. As influenza initially came into existence, authorities regularly insisted that it was just regular influenza at first, not Spanish flu. Nearly regularly, before the outbreak erupted, authorities told the nation that the worst had occurred.

This trend replicated itself over and again. Chicago gives an example of this: its advocate for public safety claimed the mayor should do 'nothing to mess with neighborhood values.' "It is our responsibility to avoid terror amongst the men worried about attacks worse than the epidemic" (Robertson, 1918).

The notion – "Fear destroys faster than sickness" – became a mantra nationwide and in town after towns. "Fear is our first opponent," *Literary Digest*, one of the largest publications in the world, advised.

In Philadelphia, when the public health commissioner closed all the schools, worship houses and other places of public gathering, the newspapers went so far as to say that this order was "not a measure to public health" and reiterated that "there was no cause for panic or alarm."

In Chicago, the death rate for all influenza patients in Cook County Hospital, not just those with pneumonia, was 39.8 percent. In Philadelphia, corpses went uncollected for days in the houses before buses, and even carts with horses were slowly driven onto the streets, and residents were ordered to carry the deceased to their houses. They were piled without coffins and buried in mass graves excavated by steam shovels in cemeteries.

This terrible split of reassurances and fact ruined the reputation of those in control. People felt they had nowhere to run to, nothing to trust, none to believe.

Society essentially relies on confidence. The society continued to disintegrate without it. Usually, America supported strangers in 1918 while somebody became sick. It was not before the pandemic. Typically, the director of the volunteers worked in one area, and irritated by repeated requests for help, was unhurt and disdainful: hundreds of women, contented to sit in the positions of angels of grace and lovely dreams, had the unfathomable pride to believe that they were able to offer a great sacrifice. Then, nobody appeared to be waking them. They were advised that there were families of which each participant becomes sick, and the children simply starve, and nobody offers them food. The mortality rate was too big, so it was always retained. This mentality still continued beyond the towns. In rural Kentucky, the Red Cross confirmed that "people die of malnutrition not because of a shortage of food but because of the fear of the healthy and are not helping the poor."

With the virus 'burden on, the internal Red Cross sources suggested that "in many parts of the country, fear and panic of influenza, like Middle Ages terror over the Black Plague, has prevailed" (The Mobilization of the American National Red Cross, 1920). Victor Vaughan, a serious scientist who did not overestablish himself, was also worried, "If the disease increases its mathematical escalation pace, humanity might easily ... wait a few weeks before the planet disappears."

Obviously, the epidemic created terror, irrespective of the acts or behavior of officials. However, the distrust of officials and the media systemically undermined morale. It magnified anxiety and transformed it into anger and panic.

It should be remembered that this fear does not appear, at least frozen, to materialize in the few instances where officials tell the facts.

One message becomes evident from this experience: it is utterly important to preserve integrity when addressing every crisis. The worst thing you can do is to offer false reassurance. If I may guess, let me assume that lying keeps knowledge so strongly that officials feel that they know more than they claim.

The Site of Origin

We can never learn with confidence that the virus crossed into a man in 1918. Throughout the 1920s and 1930s, excellent prosecutors began major searches of proof investigating the place of origin in many countries. They did not answer the question honestly. Still, as an investigator noted, they were united in agreeing that no documented outbreak in China could be "reasonably considered as the real counterpart" to the epidemic.

They considered France and the United States as the most likely sites of origin and most agreed with Macfarlane Burnet, who concluded that the evidence was "strongly evocative" that the 1918 influenza pandemic started in the United States, and that its spread was "intimately linked to war and in particular to the arrival in France of American troops."

My own work always leads me to conclude that the US was the most probable place of origin. The finding of previously discovered epidemiological proofs prompted me to create my own theory that the pandemic started in rural Kansas and brought citizens to Fort Riley today.

However, it is not really relevant if the pandemic began in France or the United States. What counts is that the pandemic had most certainly not begun in Asia.

This has important consequences for current tracking activities. If Asia's population density and its near proximity to humans and animals are especially harmful in the area, the 1918 evidence — confirming the 2003 H7N7 epidemic in Europe — proves the need for surveillance around the globe.

Anything also will be discussed in terms of tracking. A public health practitioner who earned his medical diploma in 1986 in Honduras claims he and his colleagues were told that there was little distinction between cold and influenza. He claims that medical practitioners in Central America and even other areas of the world systematically neglect flu. Clearly, if we want a sound surveillance program, doctors ought to be alert to the illness.

Data

Over the years, excellent laboratory experts have taken tremendous strides to recognize the infection and establish successful antiviral drugs along with modern vaccine technologies. Yet there is also one field in which academics remain behind —new techniques and mathematical approaches being applied to old results.

By comparison, the flooding of the Sacramento River, one of the few waterways in the world where the sole responsibility for flood management rests in the United States, are comparable. Engineers' Army Squad. The Corps has strong machines, but the Sacramento River has undergone a flood of every 100 years three times in the past ten years, which is catastrophic in California — given the reality that it sets the threshold for a flood every 100 years. The argument is not because, in 10 years, the river has reached 100 years three times. That could be described by random chance. This was even after the Corps modified the concept of a 100-year storm. A senior officer with the Corps acknowledged that the Corps did not actually have adequate evidence to determine what a 100-year flood was.

We might be in a common influenza condition. During the 20th century, we saw just three pandemics. It is not a strong foundation for constructing templates. Nonetheless, the analysis of what will happen in the United States in the event of another pandemic estimate that the death rate will decline most certainly from 89,000 to 207,000, according to the Centers for Disease Control and Prevention. Nevertheless, the true mortality rates in two of the three pandemics fall well below the range expected. One thousand nine hundred and sixty-eight fatalities have been calibrated for the population much less than the best-case scenario and in 1918 about 800% less than the worst. We still have not taken advantage of the evidence that we have. (In 1918, antibiotics potentially narrowed this difference, but the growing population of people with weakened immune systems will still offset that benefit and raise deaths.) Many conference presentations show the reality — by drawing conclusions of importance from the 1918 analyses of documents, but also from the negative side, by some assumptions about 1918, which run counter to actual data.

A detailed analysis of old data will also prove useful. Studies in 1889 (and ample evidence can be collected, probably from early pandemics too), 1918, 1957, and 1968 may inform us how it follows the same trends, which in effect allows us to improve antiviral with vaccine strategies.

The Next Pandemic

Virtually any influenza specialist claims another pandemic is almost imminent, destroying millions of persons, injuring hundreds of millions — and a virus such as 1918, or H5N1, could destroy one hundred million or more — and creating significant economic and social damage. This noise might also injure.

Despite this evidence, every laboratory investigator and every public health officer interested in the disease has two tasks: first, to do its work; secondly, to increase consciousness of the danger among political leaders. The preparatory activity needs money. We will only be appointed through the democratic party.

HOW DO VIRUSES CAUSE PANDEMICS

What Is A Virus?

Unlike a bacterial infection, genetic material can only reproduce in a cell. Most people question, "What is a virus definition?" Although trying to stay healthy in the latest Sars-cov2 epidemic. The solution to the concept of the virus is simple: it is a protein-circumcised infectious agent that includes genetic material. Viruses are also impossible to destroy while living human works. A virus wants a living thing for a long time to live. Though viruses are a living thing, what is a virus when you search for it? You will see viruses unable to live on their own for longer than a few days.

Viruses are microscopic and can't be seen when specialized medical instruments are used. The latest Sars-cov2 is one-thousandth of an eyelash's diameter, which makes it impossible to see even with a good microscope. For most viruses that can harm the human body, this is the case. When you know what a virus is made of, you also want to know its fundamental characteristic. The responses are extremely clear. Viruses are microscopic genetic material packages that reproduce in a host. They will reach the cells and wreak havoc on creation. It is extremely difficult to kill viruses.

Many of us have had the painful experience of getting drugs to make us feel better when we've been sick. It can be disappointing when the doctor says it's contagious. You may ask, "What is a viral infection?" "Viruses are difficult to kill and do not respond to antibiotics (medications that kill bacteria)." Since the latest Sars-cov2strain, finding a cure is especially difficult for physicians.

Viruses are usually much smaller tiny viruses than bacteria. They lack the ability to survive and reproduce outside a host body.

Viruses are mainly known to be the source of contagion. This prestige has undoubtedly been boosted by the frequent occurrences of disease and death. I recall the 2014 Ebola outbreak in West Africa and the 2009 H1N1/swine flu pandemic (a massive worldwide outbreak). Although such viruses are definitely rivals of scientists and doctors, others of their ilk have been influential as research tools, helping to understand the fundamental cell mechanisms, such as protein synthesis dynamics, and the viruses themselves.

Discovery

How much smaller are the most bacterial viruses? A little. A tiny more. The measles virus is nearly eight times smaller, with a diameter of 220 nanometers than the E. coli bacteria. Hepatitis is nearly 40 times smaller at 45 nm than E. coli. David R. Wessner, a biology professor at Davidson College, has offered an analogy in a 2010 paper in the journal *Nature Education*: the poliovirus, 30 nm long, is 10,000 times smaller than a grain of salt. The first vital evidence of the presence of the former was these variations in the scale between viruses and bacteria.

The conception that microorganisms, especially bacteria, may trigger disease was well known towards the end of the 19th century. Nonetheless, researchers who studied a disturbing disease of tobacco – the mosaic disease of tobacco – were quite adamant regarding the origin.

Adolf Mayer, a German chemist, and natural scientist, reported the findings of his extensive studies in 1886 in his study paper "*Concerning the Mosaic Disease of Tobacco.*" Mayer observed, infact, that when he smashed tainted leaves and squeezed the toxic juice into the veins of good tobacco plants, the disease was marked by yellowish speckling and discoloration. Mayer rightly concluded that everything that triggered the mosaic disease of tobacco was in the water. More specific outcomes, though, eluded him. Mayer was confident that what triggered the disease was infectious, but could not distinguish or classify the disease-causing agent under a microscope. He did not replicate the disease by introducing a variety of recognized bacteria into stable plants.

In 1892, a Russian student called Dmitry Ivanovsky replicated Mayer's juicing findings basically but with a change. According to an article from *Bacteriological Studies* in 1972, Ivanovsky transferred the juice from contaminated leaves through a Chamberland filter, a fairly fine filter to capture bacteria and other established microorganisms. Notwithstanding the sieve, the liquid filtrate appeared contagious, which indicated that the puzzle was a fresh piece; whatever triggered the disease was tiny enough to travel through the filter. Yet Ivanovsky also claimed that the origin of the mosaic disease of tobacco was bacterial, indicating that filtrate "produced either bacteria or a soluble toxin." Although verifying the findings of Ivanovsky, the Netherlands scientist Martinus Beijerinck claimed that the origin of tobacco mosaic illness was not a bacterial but a 'living liquid virus,' leading to the now obsolete word 'filterable virus.' It would take a few decades for us to see an infection. According to an article written in *Clinical Microbiology Reports* in 2009, the first viral with modern high-resolution technologies could be visualized after the electron microscope was invented in 1931 by German scientists Ernst Ruska and Max Knoll. Such first pictures of the tobacco mosaic virus were captured by Ruska and associates in 1939. The identification of viruses was also complete

Structure

Viruses teeter on the edge of what life is called. The main components that make up a living entity, on the one side, are the nucleic acids, DNA or RNA (any viruses may have either one or another). Viruses, on the other hand, are unable to interpret and operate on the knowledge found in these nucleic acids individually.

'A limited virus is an infection that wants to be repeated (to produce a duplicate of itself) in a host cell,' said Austin University of Texas professor Jaquelin Dudley. This is possible for viruses to generate RNA from their DNA (the so-called transcription method) and to create proteins based on the instructions contained in the RNA method. "The virus can't replicate itself outside the host as it has no complex machinery like a [host] cell does."

Once a virus is fully developed and contagious, it is considered a virion. The composition of a basic virion, according to writers of *"Natural Microbiology 4th Ed."* (University of Texas Natural Branch in Galveston, 1996), contains an internal nucleic acid nucleus enclosed by an exterior protein jar known as the capsid. Capsids inhibit the regulation and degradation of viral nucleic acids through specific host cell enzymes called nucleases. Many viruses are known as the shell as a second security sheet. This coating typically comes from the host's cell membrane, tiny stolen parts changed, and reused for use by the virus.

The DNA or RNA present in the virus heart may be single or double-stranded. This is the genome or the amount of the genetic material of a virus. Viral genomes are low in the scale, coding only for the essential proteins required for replication within a host cell, such as capside proteins, enzymes, and proteins.

Function

The main role of virology is "to transmit a genome with DNA or RNA into the host cell so that the gene can be transmitted (transcribed and translated) through the host cell," in accordance with "Natural Microbiology." Respiratory passages and open wounds may act as a virus portal. Insects also have the mode of entry. Many viruses float in an insect's saliva and enter the body of the host after the bites. According to writers of *"Molecular Cell Biology, 4th Ed"* (Garland

The Spanish Flu

Science, 2002), viruses such as these can multiply both within insect and host cells to ensure the movement between insect and host cells are smooth. Examples contain yellow and dengue fever viruses.

The viruses are then bound to the cell surfaces of the host. You do this by identifying and connecting cell surface receptors like two closed pieces of the puzzle. Many different viruses can bind to the same receiver, and a single virus may attach to multiple surface cell receivers. Although viruses use them, cell surface receptors are designed to serve the cell.

After a virus attaches to a host cell's surface, it can start moving over the host cell's exterior cover or membrane. There are a number of common entry types. HIV, an antibody infection, fuses with the membrane and is spread. The influenza virus is another enveloped virus, which is surrounded by the host. Many non-enveloped viruses, like the poliovirus, build a weak entrance path and burrow the membrane.

Viruses unleash their genomes once inside and also interrupt or hijack different parts of the cellular system. Viral genomes eventually steer host cells to generate viral proteins (many times to interrupt the production of any RNA and proteins the host cell can use). Ultimately, viruses stack the deck for themselves both within and inside the host, creating conditions for them to propagate. For, e.g., in the case of cold, a single sneeze releases, according to the molecular biology of the cell, 20 000 droplets containing rhinoviruses or new Sars-cov2particles, touching or respiring those droplets is what you need for a cold to propagate.

New discoveries

The analysis of the interactions between viruses began with the discovery of differences in size and shape, whether DNA or RNA viruses were present and in what manner. We are constantly improving our understanding of viruses and their evolution with better methods for decoding and analyzing viral genomes and the ongoing influx of new scientific evidence.

Until 1992, it was taken for granted that viruses were much smaller than bacteria with tiny genomes. That year, according to Wessner, scientists discovered a bacterial structure in a water-cooling tower. As it turned out, what they found was a very big virus called Mimivirus and not a bacterial type. The virus ranges about 750 nm and may also have the same color characteristics as gram-positive bacteria. The detection of other large viruses such as mamavirus and megavirus followed.

"The production of such massive viruses is uncertain," said Dudley, referring to them as the virus world's "elephants." "There could be degenerated cells that have become certain cell parasites (Mimiviruses invade amoeba) or more common viruses that tend to acquire additional host genes," she said. Mimiviruses, like other smaller viruses, need a cellular system from the host to generate proteins. Nevertheless, their genome also retains several genes that remain related to the translation process. Mimiviruses may have been independent cells once. Wessner reported that they probably could have gained and stored any host genes.

Such results raise new concerns and open up new areas in the study. In the future, these experiments can provide answers to fundamental questions about the nature of viruses, how they have entered their current parasite, and if viruses should be included in the life-tree.

WHY THE SECOND WAVE OF THE 1918 SPANISH FLU WAS SO DEADLY

Spanish flu's first outbreak was not especially lethal. But it came back with revenge in the fall.

The horrific severity of the influenza pandemic of 1918—called the "Italian flu "— is impossible to track. The virus infected 500 million people worldwide, killing approximately 20 million-50 million people, more than the combined number of soldiers and civilians killed during the First World War.

While the worldwide pandemic lasted two years, in the autumn of 1918, the overwhelming majority of casualties were crammed into three extremely cruel months. Historians today conclude that the catastrophic nature of the "second outbreak" of Spanish flu was triggered by a mutant virus transmitted by war troop movements.

The first appearance of Spanish flu in early March 1918 was characterized by the seasonal flu, although a very contagious and virulent strain. Some of the first examples were Albert Gitchell, a U.S. resident military chef, who was hospitalized with a 104-degree fever at Camp Funston, Missouri. The epidemic circulated exponentially among the Army's 54,000 troops. At the end of the month, 1,100 troops had been wounded, and 38 were killed during pneumonia.

As US soldiers mobilized en masse for the fight in Europe, they were bringing with them the Spanish flu. The virus spread like wildfire in England, France, Spain, and Italy throughout April and May 1918. In the spring of 1918, estimated three-quarters of the French military and as many as half of the British troops were infected. Thankfully, the virus's first outbreak was not particularly deadly, with signs such as high fever and molestation normally lasting for only three days and mortality rates comparable to seasonal flu.

How the Spanish Flu Got Its Name

Interestingly, the Spanish flu received its misnomer around this period. During World War I, Spain was neutral and did not enforce wartime restrictions on its newspapers, unlike its European neighbors. Newspapers in France, England, and the United States were not allowed to publish something that might harm the war effort, even reports that troops were sweeping a paralyzing virus. The pandemic was recognized as the Spanish flu because two of the few Spanish newspapers recorded a major influenza epidemic during the spring of 1918. The confirmed occurrence of Spanish flu fell during the summer of 1918 with optimism that the infection had stabilized by the beginning of August. It was just the quiet before the hurricane in retrospect. Somewhere in Europe, a mutant strain of Spanish influenza had grown, which had the ability, within 24 hours, of displaying the first signs of infection to destroy a perfectly healthy young man or woman.

At the end of August 1918, naval ships sailed for Plymouth, England, bringing troops unknown to treat this latest, far more lethal Spanish flu type. The second phase of the global pandemic started when such ships entered cities such as Brest in France, Boston in the United States, and Freetown in Western Africa.

James Harris, a scholar at Ohio State University who studies both infectious disease and World War 1 research said, "The massive travel of troops abroad became a significant spreader of the disease. The entire military-industrial complex of transporting more people and resources in overcrowded environments definitely played a significant part in the direction the pandemic spreads."

Virus Killed the Young, Old, and In-Between

The mortality toll from Spanish flu increased from September to November 1918. Throughout the United States alone, 195,000 People suffered from Spanish flu in October 2018. And, unlike a normal seasonal flu, the second wave of Spain's influenza showed what is known as a "W curve" – high numbers of deaths among young and old, but also a huge spike in the center, which was made of otherwise healthy 25 or 35-year-olds in their prime life.

"The medical facility was quite shocked because this atypical jump occurred in the center of the W," said Harris.

It was not only surprising that millions of good young people and women died globally, but it was also how they died. Hit by blistering fever, respiratory bleeding, and pneumonia, patients soaked in their own lungs.

Just decades later, scientists were able to explain the phenomenon, now known as "cytokine eruption." The immune system sends out signaling proteins called cytokines to facilitate beneficial immunity while the human body is invaded by a virus. But some flu strains, particularly the Spanish flu strain H1N1, may cause a dangerous immune overreaction in healthy people. The body is overwhelmed with cytokines that induce extreme inflammation and lethal deposition of fluid in the lungs.

In these situations, the severe harm to the lungs was identified by British military doctors carrying out autopsies of soldiers killed from this second wave of Spanish flu as close to the results of chemical warfare.

Lack of Quarantines Allowed Flu to Spread and Grow

Harris believes that in the autumn of 1918, the swift spread of Spanish flu was at least partly the fault of public health authorities who were unable to impose quarantines during the war. Throughout London, for example, an influential government agent named Arthur Newsholme understood that the only approach to stop the outbreak of a highly infectious illness was a complete civilian lockout. Yet he would not be in danger of paralyzing the war effort by stopping bombs and other government staff at home.

Newsholme argued, according to the Harris report, that "the unceasing fighting must explain [the] danger of transmitting illness," and urged British citizens to merely "act" through the pandemic.

A serious nursing shortage hampered public health response to the crisis in the US as thousands of nurses had been deployed in military camps and frontlines. This deficiency was exacerbated by the refusal of the American Red Cross to use trained African American nurses until the worst pandemic had passed.

Medical Science Didn't Have the Tools

However, one of the key reasons Spanish influenza took so many lives in 1918 was the inability of medicine to produce a viral vaccine. Before the 1930s, even microscopes did not perceive anything as incredibly tiny as a virus. Rather, in 1918, high-ranking medical practitioners became persuaded that the flu was attributed to a bacterium named "Pfeiffer's bacillus." A German scientist by the name of Richard Pfeiffer, following a global flu epidemic in 1890, discovered that all his sick patients became carriers of a certain type of bacteria named H. flu. As the Spanish flu pandemic struck, experts attempted to find a solution for the bacillus of Pfeiffer. Millions of dollars were spent in state-of-the-art labs to improve HT research and treatment techniques. Influenzae, naught any of it.

"This has become a fantastic diversion for medical research," Harris noted.

By December 1918, Spanish flu was the deadly second wave, but the pandemic was far from over. Throughout January 1919, a new epidemic broke out in Sydney and subsequently spread to Europe and the United States. It is claimed that after World War I peace talks in Paris in April 1919, President Woodrow Wilson was diagnosed with the Spanish flu.

The third wave mortality levels were as strong as the second, but at the end of the war in November 1918, circumstances were reduced, which enabled the disease to propagate so far and so quickly. Whilst already in millions, worldwide casualties from the third wave palpated relative to catastrophic fatalities during the second wave.

WORLD WAR ONE'S ROLE IN THE WORST EVER FLU PANDEMIC

The large 1918-19 influenza pandemic, often referred to as Spanish flu, caused approximately 50 million worldwide deaths, much more than the deaths from the fighting victims of the First World War (1914-2018). This could have consumed between 3% and 6% of the world's population.

During the early flu seasons (usually during winter), pandemic influenza was foreign to the planet, and even people prone to milder forms of influenza had limited immunity against this more virulent version of the virus. So because that occurred in pre-antibiotic days, it became possible that heavily infectious people would suffer from respiratory pneumonia, so complicating bacterial infections.

The pandemic began in January 1918 and overlapped with the war for nine months. When citizens went home, they continued. Indeed, in its scope and intensity, fighting played a major part.

A shrinking world

The First World War became a turning point in transportation. Before 1914, few citizens traveled large distances and prevented the transmission of contagious disorders, such as influenza, from one place to another and nation to another. Yes, certain rural communities were able to survive without access to many of the diseases prevalent in cities for years.

The war saw vast quantities of troops and associated staff, both within and across continents, mobilizing and fleeing, and tearing up the lives of millions of non-combatants, especially in Europe. Persons from away became more closely linked and vulnerable to every modern kind of flu than ever before.

Initially exposed to pandemic influenza, people from formerly remote areas, including Alaska or the Pacific Islands, became two times susceptible. In Western Samoa, for example, 22% of the people were destroyed, possibly because there was little preventive protection from exposure to earlier types of (seasonal) flu.

Army volunteers from a wide variety of cultures were put together to stay in near proximity in army barracks, troopships, and trench dugouts. Exposed to pandemic flu, poor residents were more prone to suffer than metropolitan people (for the same cause as the Pacific Islands and Alaskans).

Regardless of age, among those who had served in the service for long periods of time, mortality was lower. This indicates that the soldiers were slowly immunized with reactions to seasonal flu in the months and years after the induction well before the pandemic strain of flu arrived, and one or more bacterial infection which resulted in catastrophic influenza pneumonia.

New and deadly

But how can we handle the influenza pandemic of 1918? From where did it come, why was it so fatal?

They have already learn the genetic essence of the pandemic virus, along with a nuclear acid study of infectious samples from laboratories of anatomy and from corpses excavated from the Alaskan Permafrost, where Spanish flu has been separated from whole towns.

The pandemic virus has demonstrated that some gene fragments, such as those from pig and bird flu, were unique to humans in 1918. But even a novel virus with animal characteristics may have needed more research in order to circulate efficiently throughout the human community.

The dynamics of the war supported it. When individuals residing locally were contaminated, and the number of persons and viruses spread grew, the total size of the infectious population was quickly expanded.

Through the creation of several more viruses, new mutations may evolve and propagate more easily among humans. These rapidly spreading varieties may soon have rivaled the slower-growing virus types.

And they presented an even greater threat of the viral load, which overwhelmed the infected immune system and contributed to serious disease or death.

A safer time

Influenza traveled across the globe in many waves from August 1918, infecting nearly everyone. This induced disease in 20% to 50% of infected people and death in 1% to 5%.

While the pandemic influenza virus appeared to survive after 1918-19, in later years, it seemed to be less serious. That was mainly because people with the initial treatment of a limited dose of the virus had a moderate assault and then shielded themselves from any potential attack.

Furthermore, it should have prevented the spread of the most violent viruses and encouraged the spread of copies causing milder diseases through the exclusion of individuals with extreme influenza, which became normal once the pandemic became complete.

In the century after the First World War, things have improved, rendering the pandemic influenza catastrophe 1918-19 impossible to happen again. There are few enclaves in which residents are not at least partly covered from daily access to seasonal influenza or vaccine with expanded travel and changes in medical treatment.

And if a wicked new flu virus appears again, fewer populations would be vulnerable to its proliferation and development into an active pandemic epidemic. However, we already have medications for stopping their spread and managing the symptoms of serious infections easily.

THE U.S. MILITARY AND THE INFLUENZA PANDEMIC OF 1918–1919

The US combat background of World War I and the pandemic of influenza is strongly interwoven. The fighting fostered influenza in the cramped environments of military bases in the US and the Western Front trenches in Europe. During a high point of the American military's participation in the war, influenza and pneumonia sickened 20 to 40 percent in the Nation, including service forces from camp to camp and around the Atlantic. Such elevated levels of morbidity clashed with U.S. recruitment and preparation plans and rendered hundreds of thousands of military personnel ineffective. During the offensive by the American Expeditionary Forces in Meuse-Argonne, the disease redirected the requisite money from combat to transport and to look after the wounded and the dead. Throughout the battle, influenza and pneumonia destroyed more US troops and sailors than enemy arms.

In the fall of 1918, the United States army and navy medical officers were watching over the greatest outbreak in American history in camps around the world, but the tale was not fresh. Fighting and illness have been associated throughout wars in history through armies, arms, and human pathogens. The conquistadores brought disease to the New World; typhus plagued the armies of Napoleon, and typhus humiliated the US Army during the Spanish-American War. However, US armed forces and Naval staff were trained to check and sanitize water sources, vaccinate typhoid and pox soldiers, and cure or avoid other diseases. It seemed like modern bacteriology had tamed many diseases. Navy Surgeon General William C. Braised confidently claimed "the contagious diseases that once killed thousands of men, such as yellow fever, typhus, cholera, and typhoid, have all succumbed to our scientific understanding of their origins and our subsequent rational steps taken to avoid them." When the European arms race broke out of combat of 1914, the nations stunned each other and the globe with their cannons and machine guns 'fighting forces, their ships and mines, and their mustard gas.' The modern guns caused fresh, horrific casualties that took life and limb in a moment, which were gangrene wounds that could further injure and destroy. The carnage traumatized several people into a shell shock, and poison gasses smothered some so badly that nurses were unable to look for them so they could get no support. Combat diseases — especially diarrhea, dysentery, and typhus of the soldiers — flourished, and the trenches provided new diseases, such as the "trench foot," an illness owing to the wearing of sodium boots and the end of the days in water and dirt, as well as the "trench flu," a deteriorating body fog.

Then, in the fourth awful year of the war, when the US Expeditionary Forces (AEF) took on military strength and planned their first significant offensive against the Germans, the flu hit. By the most optimistic calculation of the War Department, 26 percent of the army, of over one million soldiers, sickened with flu, murdered almost

30,000 civilians before they had entered France. In 1918, the Army suffered incredibly to influenza. They had to enlist about 8,743,102 people on both sides of the Atlantic. The Navy reported 5,027 deaths and more than 106,000 hospital visits of 600,000 people because of influenza and pneumonia, yet Braised took the illness rate closer to 40 percent, despite the vast amount of mild cases never registered.

The medical services of the Army and Navy may have tamed typhus, but more troops, seafarers, and Marines would fall to influenza and pneumonia than would perish in the Great War's global battlegrounds. The influenza outbreak in the military is sometimes forgotten in the chronological narrative of the Greater War, which corresponds with the last fighting and the Armistice as a coda for this four-year terror. Nevertheless, reviewing news records from the war room and the Navy room shows that the fighting and the outbreak have become intertwined. World War I and influenza have cooperated: war-fueled fever by developing environments in France's trenches, which some epidemiologists claim also helped the flu virus to develop into a global killer. In addition, influenza dominated the war effort by rendering the Army and Navy equipment, workforce, and precious human time and energy inefficient and disruptive. Many measures, such as crowd reduction and quarantines to contain the disease,were also hampered by war requirements. The flu outbreak in the US military also offers a cautionary account of war's ability to transform the health atmosphere and the capacity of illness to affect fighting.

Going To War

At first, the United States held back from the murder in Europe, as many Americans felt that it was not their task. But President Wilson abandoned neutrality and asked the Congress to make a declaration of war under increasing pressure from Britain and France and irritated by German U- attacks that endangered American commerce and security and the revelations on the Zimmermann Telegram that Germany urged Mexico to attack the US.

When producers and suppliers exported grain and military equipment to the warring countries, the US economy had already been thriving. The USA now established its own unit, helping to overpower the enemy and bring on the armistice of 11 November 1918. Congress soon adopted a list, with over 4,600 list Selective Service boards examining 10 million people to select the most appropriate suited troops and sailors. The population expanded to more than 4,7 million from just 378,000 in April 1917, including a population of 4,1 million and a fleet of 600,000. Seventy-two percent of the forces enlisted and the military population, reflected the ethnically diverse and racially separated society of the country. It is known that about 20 percent of the force was foreign-born, and the soldiers spoke 46 languages, about 5,700 were Mexican immigrants, and 12,500 were Americans. There were more than 400,000 African Americans in the force, some from two black-fighting units but more from agriculture. Just 5,300 Black sailors were hired by the Navy and classified as cooks and stewards.

The U.S. Military And The Influenza Pandemic Of 1918–1919

The mobilization of war drew millions of people to military establishments and dispersed the military across the world. The Armed Forces and the Navy also extended current facilities and conducted recruitment programs with various civic groups to educate and support these people. Across both nations, military bases, arsenals, airfields, and equipment depots sprouted up. In the fall of 1917, the Army started preparing soldiers in 32 large camps of 25,000 to 55,000 troops each. Soldiers were also sent to different advanced field training centers such as Camp Knox, Kentucky, Camp Benjamin Harrison railway activities at Indianapolis, combat infrastructure at Camp Forrest, Georgia, and instruction in the medical unit at Camp Crane, Pennsylvania. The War Division also maintained 40 aviator testing airfields and ten transport and debarkation centers. The Navy increased its capability to over 100,000 stations on both sides, the Gulf of Mexico and Lake Michigan from 6,000 recruiters, as well as advanced educational facilities such as the Columbia University Navy Gas Engine School and Cloud Fire Aviation School in New York. Throughout the summer of 1918, the War Department set up, in addition to the boot centers, the Student Army Training Corps (SATC), designed to raise the Reserve Officers Training Corps (ROTC) and to discourage war mobilization from emptying higher education institutions. The system has educated more than 500 colleges and universities and received professional training in areas such as automobile mechanics and electronics. Through the Armistice, nearly 158,000 young people enrolled in SATC programs. The proliferation of military organizations created a global network of young adults who can and should fly via influenza.

When the nation expanded, the Medical Department of the Army was up to its needs. Army practice was more comparable to public health practice (which treated vast populations) than private medicine. Line officers were generally less worried about who was ill or on leave than who they should submit to battle. It was considered the "successful" limit — how many people should function and battle in a given unit. Therefore, medical officers sought to preserve as small as possible the inadequate levels and evaluated their performance objectively rather than actual patient treatment. The Army Medical Department monitored illness every day, week, month, and year in barracks, military forces, labor battalions, ports, and ships and contrasted it with people, early wars, and other armies. Army Health also mixed the traditional safe water and fresh air treatment paradigm with modern public safety strategies to teach troops about preserving wellness and avoiding disease. General surgeon of the Army, William C. Gorgas, came from a healthy tradition and stressed good food, clean water, fresh air, and no crowds, but like other progressive army members, he saw the Army as an opportunity to introduce young men to middle-class values, such as good hygiene.

The Health Department also expanded the medical capacity from 9,500 to 120,000 in the United States alone to support the increasing army. The Red Cross helped attract qualified nurses and coordinated emergency companies and 50 clinics, each with 1000 beds, from American medical universities. In the end, 30 500 Military Personnel, 21 500 nurses – 350 African American doctors but not black nurses – and 264 000 people were enrolled in the Army Medical Corps. There were about 3,000 military staff, 1,700 nurses, and 11,000 people serving in the Navy Department of Medicine and Surgery. As one civil official for public safety stated with about 30% of the US military staff, "There have been parts of the world completely robbed of clinicians." Thus, during a civil disorder pandemic, 'the overwhelming majority of medical and nursing services available were either in the military or naval, rendering the resources accessible. Although about 55,000 Marines were deployed for the AEF, the Navy's duties included patrolling vessels, wading hostile mines, escorting soldiers and supply ships around the Atlantic, and digging toward the German Navy in the North Sea. In the US, mobilization started gradually, and the AEF had fewer than 400,000 in Europe a year after the declaration of war. Nevertheless, by May 1918, hundreds of thousands of troops crossed the Atlantic every month in order to create a military power of two million by November. It was one of the major successes of the First World War, and it demonstrated the strength of the US government and the economy. Yet such a victory still faced a risk, as the boys did not ride alone when driving "over there."

A Lethal Virus

Influenza swept through the Atlantic with American soldiers, and when it erupted in Europe and the United States in late August and September, medical officers were on the frontlines of an outbreak more than anything they had ever previously witnessed or expected. Some of the country's most experienced and trained doctors had only entered the armed service recently. They tried their best to rescue those who were afflicted by influenza but could do nothing more than include palliative treatment with food, rest, and a gentle diet.

One of the tragedies of the influenza outbreak was that, by the 1910s, a significant number of research and epidemiological methods in the medical profession were utilized to recognize the existence and severity of the losses done by influenza and pneumonia and could not have the requisite resources to fight them effectively. Although virology did not arise until the 1930s, doctors were able to recognize several of the bacteria causing lethal pneumonia to destroy their patients but could do nothing to stop the infections without antibiotics. So several medical officers reported what they witnessed as the disease reached their villages, clinics, aircraft, ports, or units as though to be trying to identify something they could not monitor. They carried out experiments and conducted autopsies, reported their experimental and clinical results, measured morbidity and mortality levels over time and with other groups, and sought to stay healthy. They sent extensive letters to their bosses and reported numerous influenza publications from 1918–1919. These papers and analyses included some of the most detailed documentation on the pandemic, educating civil and military scholars of their attempts to explain what sparked the disease and the pervasive devastation for years after the outbreak.

As they examined the outbreak of influenza, military medical staff soon realized that the first phase of the pandemic had swept through several U.S. training centers in spring 1918. In March, April, or May, 14 of the largest training camps announced influenza outbreaks, and some sick troops brought the virus to France by sea. Late spring and summer, all the armies of Europe, including the AEF, were visited by influenza, but because the military was frequently influenced and few patients were severely ill, there was no alarm from medical officers. Yet others saw fresh, deadly influenza appear in the late summer.

Captain Alan M. Chesney, a medical officer at Valdahon AEF hospital, an artillery training camp behind France's front lines, reported from his viewpoint the production of virulent influenza. A specialist who eventually became Dean of the Johns Hopkins School of Medicine, Chesney, stated that three separate infantry brigades of 4,000 people took up the position, "and every three or four weeks, the composition of the post varied dramatically." Thus the epidemic's past "was calculated to be various periods in accordance with the diverse brigades." During the second period, 27 July to 23 August, 200 members of the 58th Artillery Brigade, 6.5 percent, became sick. None were killed, but the epidemic was too severe for the next division to scrub the barracks, or to wash the doors before going back. In the third step of Chesney, from 23 August to 8 November, about one-third of the 6th Artillery Division, 1636 men, contracted the flu, and 151 died amid this measure. Chesney argued that "these repeated outbreaks became increasingly more serious in nature and extent, due to the enhanced virulence of the causative agent."

Medical officers like Chesney needed clean barracks and were nervous about crowding. Surgeon General Gorgas also suggested that the army would have 60 square feet of housing per male, although not always. As Gorgas once said to a training camp director, 'We know very well that we can completely manage pneumonia if you can stop crowding people, but it is not possible to eliminate this crowding in military existence.' The Medical Department had also reported that 'there is a certain association between the degree of crowding and the amount of respiratory infection.' Evolutionary biologist Paul Ewald has concluded that trench fighting and cramped environments allowed a highly violent and lethal influenza virus to obtain human protection. When troops became wounded in the trenches, the military removed them from the front lines and substituted them with good men. This cycle continually put the virus into touch with new hosts — young, stable soldiers among which it can adjust and replicate without the possibility of burning out. According to the Navy paper, "it's fair to suppose that extreme influenza in August spread from French, Spanish and Portugal's seaports to the North, South Africa, the US, and South America." Influenza 1918 was a trench war commodity, as Chesney and Ewald indicated, and the flu which affected the 6th Valdahon Artillery should move to Valdahon.

Influenza In The Camps

Braised pointed to the beginning of the disease in the United States at the Commonwealth Pier in Boston on Tuesday 27 August 1918 when 'three cases of influenza were admitted on a sick list.' The next day, 8 cases were registered, and, on 29 August, 58 cases were recorded, 15 were sent to the United States as ill. Within 48 hours, three medical officers who had seen the patients also fell ill. Influenza reached civilians in Boston, and on September 8, they arrived in the army camp of Devens "completely unheralded" outside the town. Within ten days, thousands of injured trainees were exhausted in the base hospital and regimental diseases.

Gorgas assigned his finest epidemiologists to study Camp Devens. His staff included Victor C. Vaughan, Dean of the University of Michigan School of Medicine and Head of the General Office of Communicable Disease (COD) of the Surgeon; William Henry Welch, Johns Hopkins renowned pathologist; and Rufus Cole, Rockefeller Institute's respiratory disease specialist. We considered the medical condition "severe," and we proposed 16 disease prevention steps, the most drastic being halting transport to or from Devens before the epidemic had passed. Camp Devens autopsy practitioners identified influenza pathology as unusual, with "intense coughing and bleeding" characteristics of the lungs. Cole and Welch experienced one such operation, and Cole agreed, "There must be a different sort of virus or disease," Welch "walked away with a bloated blue lung, with a sticky, spummy, shapeless surface[and] was agitated and anxious." Cole said, "It was not shocking that the rest of us were upset, but I was surprised to see that the occurrence at least was briefly too intense." A group of substitute troops went out from Devens to Camp Upton, Long Island, to carry influenza with them, before any travel restriction could be enforced. Health officers at Upton announced that on 13 September 1918, they arrived "abruptly" with 38 referrals to hospital, accompanied by 86 the next day and the next, 193. Hospital admissions peaked at 483 on 4 October, and 6131 people were sent to the influenza hospital within 40 days. Many of them acquired pneumonia so quickly that physicians actually treated it by watching the patient instead of listening to the lungs. "The guy seemed depressed and indicated a severe condition," he read, "his face sometimes became cyanotic, often ashy, sometimes only trapped. He didn't show anxiety or discomfort. When his feelings became coherent, he displayed a euphoria or an unusual awareness of his illness that especially characterized the disease's advanced stages." Private James Downs arrived at the hospital with a fever of 104 degrees on 23 September and died three days later. A pathologist from the army sliced off a portion of the lung and submitted it to the American Army Museum with an indication of injury to young soldiers from influenza. When they crossed 900 patients in the pneumonia ward of Camp Upton, the medical officers witnessed "the terror of the terrifying sight of the hopelessly sick and dying and the size of the cataclysm of the massively impaired young soldiers prepared to face another threat, but without support, before that "sinister one." Naomi Barnett of Brockton, Massachusetts, had driven to Upton, after she heard that he was sick, to look after her fiancée Jacob Julian. They planned to marry until he left for office in France, but two days after he arrived at the village, the young woman died of pneumonia. Thirty minutes later, her husband died. "Relatives," the local daily record, "are preparing a double burial in Brockton." The hospital equipped patients with 100 square feet of floor space, different sleeping clothes and fitted facial masks, in order to contain influenza and pneumonia in the area. As the pneumonia spread, medical officers even sprayed the mouths and throats of 800 safe people with dichloramine T solutions regularly as a prevention measure, however, when comparing their flu rate to 800 untreated people they were frustrated to find that "... the incidence of both classes was similar for a period of twenty days."

As medical officers scaled their outbreak, influenza spread west and south and landed at Camp Grant, Illinois, with 70 hospital admissions on Saturday 21 September 1918. "The encounter was so abrupt and shocking that every officer, every man and every nurse was most enthusiastic and cooperated to cope with the emergency," one author reported. Hospital admissions rose to 194, then to 370, then to 492, and on September 29, they were up to 788 admissions. Hospital officials forced all the officers to depart, turned the cassettes into hospital wards, and increased hospital space with "extreme effort" in six days from "10 vacant beds to an accommodation capacity of 4,102 beds." The hospital laboratory used nearby civilian equipment for specimen processing. Patients with conjunctivitis, influenza disease, ears, nose, and throat were seen in the field by ophthalmologists who saw patients with other adverse secondary infections. If people were seriously ill, camp officers issued "risk" or "death" telegrams to families and friends, but then they had so many callbacks, telegrams, and guests that they had to create a separate medical tent as an intelligence center. Health workers were spared. Among the 81 military officers, 11 were killed, and three civilians and three army nurses were wounded. The crisis even prompted a prohibition on black nurses by the Medical Department, which appointed Camp Grant African American nurses to care for patients. However, the women had to wait before new accommodation could be installed.

Ten days after the outbreak, hospital admissions begun to fall, but pneumonia slowed, and the average death toll at Camp Grant was starting to rise. On October 1, with 14 suicides, it hit double amounts, then 30 the next day, 46 the next, and 76 on October 4. The mortuary was only planned for four deaths a day. On Friday, October 4, authorities arranged with local companies to take bodies to a mortuary camp for $50 each, but when someone produced a flatbed truck for the disposal of the deceased, the military immediately issued more dignified locked vehicles. On October 5, the number of fatalities exceeded 100 and, on October 6, hit a horrific peak of 117. The last day the death count of Camp Grant reached 100 was October 9, but its commander was too late to crash. As influenza struck, Col. Charles B. Hagadorn, a West Point graduate and career officer in the Russian and Panamanian Canal Areas, served as the director of the base. While the plague and mortality rate at Camp Grant was not higher than and greater than any other prisons, fellow officers later told the reporters that the outbreak was exacerbated by Hagadorn. Troubled by the death of more than 500 soldiers under his orders, he committed suicide with a gun fired at the head on October 7. As a result, 10,713 influenza patients were casualties at Camp Grant; 1,060 at them lived among a community of 40,000.

Throughout the country, medical personnel noted the speed with which each camp was affected by the epidemic, reaching its highest number of cases within ten days. Through the reports of The Camp Dodger, the weekly Camp Dodge, Iowa, which was tracking the outbreak, we can see the high rate of the influenza assaults. The first reference of Flu was noted on 29 September. It was first given 'Dodge Fights Spain's' Flu'; on the 4th of October. Quarantine was enforced with total cases around 1500. The following week the outbreak subsided, there were fewer new cases; mortality rate also crashed. The following week was full of joy as the news came that the outbreak has ended. Whilst Camp Dodge had one of the worst military camp reports with over 13,700 medical visits and 700 fatalities; the outbreak passed with a low death rate.

The Spanish Flu

HOW THE 1918 PANDEMIC FRAYED SOCIAL BONDS: STORY

The influenza pandemic has done long-term disruption to connections with several American societies. Can the distrust be avoided?

When Seattle authorities declared a town-wide lock-down, the 15-year old Violet Harris was relieved she didn't have to go to school anymore. "Well done, nice idea? I'm going to say it is!" She read her book, along with *USA Today*. "The only thing in my atmosphere is that the board of the [school] should incorporate the days that have gone by before the end of the year." She couldn't leave her house for hours as she sewed a dress for school before she reopened and tried new recipes in the local paper and created an especially awful sample of fudge, half of which was thrown off. This appears like she really was completely conscious of the situation after she got the shocking report that her closest mate, Rena was ill with the Spanish Flu. The two talked on the phone one week later after Rena had healed. "I told [Rena] how influenza feels, and she replied, 'Don't get it.'" Because history tends to replicate itself, it's shows that the human condition is fairly unchanged. I witnessed an unsettling spark of remembrance while reading journal papers and diaries published during the influenza pandemic of 1918. The grim comments, nervous chuckles, and respiratory uncertainty showed me I was witnessing people deal with their life under quarantine by thinking of the situation on Twitter over the last few weeks. Despite many parallels with the current scenario, the lockout in 1918 was also even lonelier than it is now. In the early 20th century, without the many networking innovations that enabled us to keep in touch with friends and family, Americans confronted the abrupt lack of close community relations, an event that, for many, also overweighed the fear of a deadly and infectious disease.

When hospitals were locked up with patients, and American cities put in quarantine, several people alternated between fear and pleasantness; for moments they panicked about the pandemic, and in other moment laughed about it. The order allowing Seattle people to wear masks in public entertained Harris in particular. She wrote, "People are going to look funny — like ghosts." She drew masks in front of her diary and pasted them into an article about the latest face mask styles.

Most citizens soon become angry about the loneliness pitfalls. "The Spanish flu, we were quarantined, and everyone is crazy," reads a letter from a soldier posted in South Carolina. Another soldier was upset that the isolation stopped him from delivering a Christmas gift to his father. Health Commissioner Max Starkloff announced in St. Louis that colleges, film studios, bars, and, perhaps, devastatingly, outdoor athletic activities would be shut down. "Influenza is affecting football here," the *St. Louis Globe-Democrat* argued. 'Health Department interventions to cause the players considerable pain.' *St. Louis Post-Dispatch* devoted article after article to the flu: 'Quarantine could continue for four weeks; football set back,' read the headline version. "Soccer games are now off. The Spanish 'flu' has put a damper on the gridiron," another student noted.

In the early period of the epidemic, citizens became increasingly upset with the way public safety interventions disrupted their everyday habits, whether they wouldn't or couldn't expect the more serious effects of the epidemic. In certain areas, though, as the death rate started to increase, there was a panic and a bleak influence on human relationships.

Because quarantine was contained, the pandemic of 1918 was mostly secret. Unable to count on friends and family for assistance, residents in houses with shuttered windows faced the crisis alone. Harris writes in her journal, "I sat all day and didn't even go to Rena's." "Mom doesn't want us to move farther than we should."

Such human feelings of isolation exacerbated the once-strong group ties in certain situations. "People were afraid to speak to each other," said Daniel Tonkel, a flu victim, during a 1997 PBS *American Experience* segment. "It was like don't breathe on my face; don't look at me; because you can give me the infection, and you never know who the next victim is," John M. Barry, author of *The Great Influenza*, told me that feelings of loneliness and mistrust intensified throughout the pandemic, especially in places like offices/organization. "Culture relies heavily on faith when you get to it, and without it, there is a resentment that runs through society," he said. "You only had yourself because you didn't have anyone to run to." In his book, Barry described the stories of families starving to death because others hated too much to bring them food. He tells me, "that you want society and family and neighborhood to feel strong enough to overcome this," not just in towns, but also in rural communities. In an interview in 1980, Glenn Hollar described the way in which social connections split in his home town of North Carolina. "There would be crowds in your room to holler and look up and see if you were still living." By December 1918, the number of new cases started to taper off, and American society began to return to normal slowly. ("The first time the nation takes a closer look at football in 1918, when the ban lifts, tomorrow," read the headline in the post-expedition of St. Louis.) However, the singular nature of the outbreak affected the way it was commemorated. The public attention quickly moved toward the end of the First World War, weakening the cathartic practices that cultures need to resolve mutual traumas. In the decades after the outbreak, the flu became stuck in the memories of men, remembered but still not addressed. American author John Dos Passos, who observed the disease on a soldier, never explained the encounter. "It never got much publicity, but it was there beneath the water," said Barry.

More than 80 years later, Thomas Mullen authored *The Last Town on Earth*, a fictitious 1918 flu story. In an interview after the book was published, Mullen spoke about 'the memories of survivors of flu in 1918,' which rapidly led to the very erasure of those memories.' Historian Alfred W. Crosby considered that the pandemic was 'America's forgetful.' In many ways, the loneliness and suspicion caused by the flu continued to pervade American society subtly. For others, something appeared to have been forever missing. "There weren't as many friendly people as before," said John Delano, a native of New Haven, Connecticut, in 1997. "They didn't visit each other; they brought food in, they always had groups. The area has shifted. Things shifted. We transformed." Yet Barry told me that this was not the case everywhere. Through his study, he noticed that local leadership talked frankly about the possibility of influenza in neighborhoods. "There was certainly a lot of apprehensions… but you did not seem to see the kind of disintegration that happened elsewhere," he said. He claims in his book that in communities where progressive public health officials showed strong leadership, people held confidence.

For one, Seattle Health Commissioner J. S. McBride implemented concrete public-health policies immediately and also donated his resources to an emergency department. In November 1918, he commended Seattle's citizens for "their cooperation with us in controlling the dramatic, though important, influenza epidemic order." McBride's behavior may have helped Seattleites like Violet Harris to recall the outbreak as a little dull.

The public meeting spaces in Seattle eventually reopened for the company following six weeks of the lockout. "This week school opens," wrote Harris in her diary. "Friday! Friday! Have you ever done so? As if they hadn't been able to sit until Tuesday!"

WEAR A MASK AND SAVE YOUR LIFE: THE 1918 FLU PANDEMIC

The pandemic of influenza of 1918 was a truly plausible pandemic, which impacted not only major population centers but also the most remote communities in the Pacific and far north of Inuit.

Any 500 million people can, at any stage, have been contaminated with 675,000 deaths alone in the United States. More citizens globally were destroyed by influenza than by World War I, a parallel, twice as long globally battle as the pandemic.

The battle, moreover, led to the widespread dissemination of the disease. War situations and troop activities around the Atlantic and across conflict areas help spread influenza all around the globe.

The disease's first occurrence in the US was in the spring of 1918, but its symptoms were mostly moderate and less serious than the norm.

Not until the fall would the epidemic deliver its most deadly strike – most of the reported 20-100 million deaths in October and November took place in a few week's time.

While medicine had taken significant strides with the invention of germ theory since the end of the 19th century, doctors and scientists remained impotent to combat influenza because of its rapidly changing existence. Instead, the responses centered on limiting its dissemination. One of the most common pieces of advice was to wear a mask.

The severity of the epidemic triggered widespread hysteria. Churches and schools were closed, while the remaining open businesses and utilities suffered from human resources shortages. Too frightened to go out in public, citizens segregated themselves, making the streets nearly bare.

After traveling 12 miles without seeing a single car, a medical student in usually busy Philadelphia remembered that "the city life has almost ended." The extreme isolation was regretted by a depressed medical community. In the event of the desperation of more people, the Director of Philadelphia's Emergency Aid said bitterly: "There are households in which children are actually hungry because no one provides them anything. The mortality rate is too big, and they still hang off." The shipbuilders who were vital to the fighting were among those who remained behind. At L.H. Shattuck Co. in New Hampshire, just 54% of its workers appeared and 41% at the Groton Iron Works in Connecticut.

There were also people on the front and wanted soldiers impacted. One of the more troubling features of grip in 1918 was its propensity to threaten young people who were previously safe. Previous influenza outbreaks ravaged mostly the aged and very young, but the strain of 1918 affected many who might have been on the front if not for illness, and were in the first place.

In early 1919, the third wave began and continued through the season, not as catastrophic as fall, but it brought severe disease and death. Finally, the outbreak ended in the summer of 1919. Scientists now recognize that it was triggered by an H1N1 virus, which had persisted for the past two years as a seasonal infection.

The Spanish Flu

ANALYSIS: SPANISH FLU PANDEMIC PROVES SOCIAL DISTANCING WORKS

People begin the second month of home social isolation, lawmakers and other leaders in public safety discuss how long civic hearings continue to be postponed. Others challenge that long-term isolation is still appropriate in order to avoid the spread of coronavirus disease in 2019 (cov-2).

Stefan E. Pambuccian, MD, MIAC, a Professor and Vice President of the Department of Pathology and Experimental Medicine in Loyola University, Chicago's Stritch School of Medicine, is attempting to address these questions in a recent paper in the *Journal of the American Society of Cytopathology*, which is the basis for the "Spanish influenza" pandemic of 1918-1919.

Briefly, his answer to if social distance works is yes.

"The more strict the regime of exclusion, the greater the risk of mortality," Pambuccian said in a media statement.

The pandemic of 1918-1919 wound up murdering nearly 50 million people globally and about 675,000 in the United States. This is given the fact that many nations, including the U.S., had banned broad public gatherings, canceled classes, and in some cases, needed helmets and other safety gear. As is today, though, Pambuccian said that part of the issue was that measures were not standardized.

"These steps were not enforced or universally adopted in various cities in the same period or for the same period," he reported.

Pambuccian examined current research literature on the past pandemic and contrasted it with established evidence and programs related to the present pandemic.

Cities such as San Francisco, St. Louis, Milwaukee, and Kansas were vigilant with their protective steps, writes Pambuccian, and their swift intervention is believed to decrease the transmitting risk by as much as 30-5%. Peak mortality and overall mortality were both smaller.

"The amount of time these measurements of 'private isolation' were retained was associated with a reduced overall mortality burden," he notes. "While we have not yet provided a proven successful treatment or vaccine protection for this coronavirus, and the environment is a very different place from 100 years ago, the efficacy of the interventions implemented during the pandemic of 1918-19 provides us with the belief that the new steps would still restrict the impact of the SARS-CoV-2 pandemic." Pambuccian acknowledged that several concerns remain about the emerging epidemic and that thus health practitioners will be especially vigilant and accessible for new knowledge.

In his article, Pambuccian, a cytologist, often discusses measures in the cytology laboratory to reduce the danger associated with the SARS-CoV-2 virus.

Many of these steps reflect the work of all health care personnel, such as ensuring that the staff meets needs, and ensuring that employees take proper precautions to protect themselves and limit the risk of transmission when the worker becomes ill. From a diagnostic point of view, the cytology laboratory is primarily capable of extracting potentially contradictory facts.

"In a patient with established COVID-19, the function of the cytology laboratory is restricted," he wrote. "The function of the cytological lab in SARS is specifically linked to the prevention of superimposed sputum and other respiratory infections." Pambuccian also stated that laboratory personnel is responsible for keeping up with the constantly changing condition, including adopting the current recommendations from the American Diseased Control and Prevention Centers and the World Healing Group.

LOOKING BACK AT THE LAWS THAT CAME WITH THE 1918 SPANISH FLU PANDEMIC

A run on advanced surgical masks designed to remove the virus has contributed to shortages in some regions. Cloth masks are just as hard to buy as soap, hand sanitizer, and toilet paper at the nearest drug shop.

The Injury Control and Prevention Centers do not allow safe individuals to use masks. The majority of patients are not strong enough to flush out infectious viruses anyway, and the use of actual antiviral masks has possibly compromised health workers, causing them to rely on those who are less successful when handling infected patients.

This shows how much had improved since the Spanish flu pandemic a century ago when masks became mandatory in those years. On 22 Nov. 1918, *Variation* announced that health officials in several cities had requested them to be worn in every location, including stores, businesses, theaters, and churches before beginning the Quarantine General. Indianapolis gave a directive to "use fabric masks exclusively in all public areas" until it was agreed to shut down industries. Back then, in some quarters, it was evident that masks were a half step that was not very effective.

Even after the quarantine was abolished, however, health authorities in some cities demanded: "all patrons wear masks." Theater managers in Los Angeles debated whether to reopen their premises after they lifted the quarantine due to the continued restrictions, "preferring to wait until the mask wear order was dispensed with."

Movie shoots hadn't been subject to commands. On 14 Feb. 1919, near the end of the terrifying second influenza outbreak, *Variety* announced that the actress Shirley Mason and producer Walter Edwards spent the night "in jail in Pasadena when they failed to comply with the legislation requiring masks to be carried during an influenza epidemic."

Throughout 1919, Mason and Edwards collaborated together on two two-reel comedies. The tale is lost as they were shut down, but the two names match the calamitous times: "The Rescue Hero" and "The Last Close-Up."

ECONOMIC EFFECTS OF THE 1918 INFLUENZA PANDEMIC

As stated earlier, the lack of economic knowledge is the greatest drawback to becoming informed of the economic consequences of influenza 1918. Any research experiments analyze the economic impact of the pandemic using accessible evidence, and these findings are analyzed later. However, in spite of the general shortage of financial evidence, print media are now accessible as a source of knowledge on (some) economic consequences of the 1918 pandemic.

Newspapers in the Little Rock and Memphis Eighth Federal Reserve District distributed in the fall of 1918 have been reviewed in order to collect details on the impact of the pandemic of influenza in these towns. Collecting anecdotal reports from particular communities will provide a fairly accurate summary of the pandemic's overall consequences.

In 1918, these general results may be used to extrapolate to the potential economic consequences of a global pandemic.

The 1918 Influenza Pandemic in the News

This involves names and reproduction of publications in the Eighth Federal Reservation District in two newspapers: *The Arkansas Gazette* (Little Rock) and *The Consumer Appeal* (Memphis).

In these magazines, as in many publications (St Louis as Louisville, for instance), stories reporting the amount of influenza sick or dead almost regularly emerged. Articles on closings of synagogue, school, and theatre, as well as questionable treatments and solutions to influenza, were published regularly.

However, there were much fewer frequent studies documenting the impact of influenza on the local economies. The following are some articles which appeared in the autumn of 1918 and addressed the economic effects of influenza.

Little Rock, Ark.

"How Influenza Affects Business." *The Arkansas Gazette*, Oct. 19, 1918, page 4.

- Little Rock merchants claim their market has decreased by 40 percent. Others predict a 70 percent fall.
- The retail grocery business has been reduced by one-third.
- There is a department store that has a daily business of $15,000 ($200,265 in 2006 dollars).
- Bed rest is emphasized in influenza treatment. As a consequence, competition for tents, mattresses, and springs has increased.
- Little Rock firms lose an amount of $10,000 a day ($133,500 in 2006). That is a complete failure, not a drop in the industry,

which may be caused by a rise in revenue at the conclusion of the quarantine period. Any products can not be marketed later.

- The only enterprise in Little Rock with a rise in sales is the drugstore

Memphis, Tenn. "Influenza Crippling Memphis Industries."

The Commercial Appeal, Oct. 5, 1918, page 7.

- Doctors say that they are too busy battling the epidemic to record the number of patients and have no time to focus on certain items.

- Chemical plants operate at a significant disadvantage. All of them had even become deprived of assistance because of the call.

- For the nearly 400 people employed in the Memphis Street Railway's transport service, 124 were incapacitated yesterday. This operation has been curtailed.

- More than one hundred operators absent from their posts are registered by the Cumberland Telephone Co. The telecommunications provider ordered the elimination of unwanted calls.

"The Commercial Appeal of Tennessee Mines That Shut Down", 18 Oct. 1918, p. 12.

- Fifty percent decrease in coal mining operators' revenue.

- Mines around East Tennessee and southern Kentucky are set to shut owing to the outbreak in the mining camps.

- Coalfield, Tennessee, has "just 2 percent of good residents for a community of 500 residents."

Survey of Economic Research

One study report explores the immediate (short-run) impact of influenza mortality on incomes from 1914 to 1919 in U.S. cities and states.

The paper's testable argument is that influenza death had a direct influence on wages in the US manufacturing sector during and shortly after influenza 1918. The theory is based on a basic labor-market economic model: a decrease in the availability of factory employees as a consequence of influenza deaths should have initially decreased the availability of industrial labor, boosted the gross output of labor, income per employee, thus raising real incomes. In the short term, labor mobility in cities and states is likely to prevent income equalization across the economy, and it is doubtful that there has been a switch away from relatively expensive labor for money.

The empirical results backed the theory that cities and states with higher mortality rates of influenza reported increased production incomes between 1914 and 1919.

Another research analyzed state income development using a common approach for the decade after the influenza pandemic. In their unfinished report, the writers suggested that further influenza deaths per year should have boosted per population development levels after the pandemic. Essentially, higher influenza death levels should have culminated in larger cost gains per job, thus more job production and higher wages after the pandemic. The authors considered a favorable and statistically meaningful association between state-wide influenza mortality levels and resulting state per capita revenue development using state personal revenue figures of 1919-1921 and 1930.

The long-term effect of 1918 influenza was examined in a recent paper. The analyst concluded that influenza exposure to utero has negative economic consequences for people later in life. The research was undertaken after the analysis of data showing that pregnant mothers subjected to influenza in 1918 carried into life infants that had significant medical issues, such as autism, diabetes, and stroke. The author hypothesizes that the health benefits of a person are directly linked to human resources and efficiency and thus, incomes and revenues.

The investigator observed that samples in utero, utilizing decennial census statistics from 1960 to 1980, had decreased educational performance, higher levels of physical injury, and poorer wages after the 1918 pandemic. In fact, if they were in utero during the pandemic "(m)en and women display substantial and persistent declines in education attainment. The offspring with contaminated mothers have a 15% reduced chance with graduation from high school. Men's salaries were 5-9% lower owing to illness."

Some data suggests that the 1918 influenza pandemic had short-term economic implications. Several corporations, especially those in the service and entertainment sectors, reported double-digit sales declines. Many firms investing in wellness goods saw sales rise. Some scholarly literature indicates that the flu pandemic of 1918 triggered labor shortages, which resulted in higher (at least temporary) salaries for the workforce, but no fair claim could be made that the gains were greater than the cost of the massive loss of life and economic activity.

Evidence also indicates that the 1918 influenza triggered a decline in human resources after the pandemic, thereby having an effect on economic practices decades after the pandemic.

Implications for a Modern-day Pandemic

The potential financial risk and death tolls discussed at the outset of this study from a global influenza pandemic in the United States indicate an eventual expense of many hundred billion dollars to hundreds of thousands or several million lives. In two influential reports on the 1918 influenza pandemic, the details provided in this article and the knowledge given is still used to devise a list of potential economic impacts of a contemporary influenza pandemic and alternative ways to minimize the intensity of any hypothetical pandemic:

- Given the positive correlation between population density and influenza mortality, the mortality rate is likely to be higher in cities than in rural areas. However, in contrast to 1918, urban and rural areas are more integrated today — the mortality gap between cities and rural areas may be minimized. Likewise, a higher proportion of the US populace is today known as metropolitan (approximately 80%) than the US populace at the height of the pandemic (51% in 1920).

• Non-White populations as a whole are more prone to die as nearly 90 percent of non-Whites reside in metropolitan environments (compared to about 77 percent of whites). It tends to do with lower-class individuals being likely to die — the mean income of non-White (excluding Asians) is small ($30,858 of 2005) relative to white ($50,784 in 2005) families. Similarly, only 10% of White citizens were below the threshold of deprivation in 2005 compared with over 20% of specific ethnic groups (with the exception of Asians).

• Urban sites are expected, on average, to have greater access to standard physical health services, but almost 19% of the metropolitan population of the United States may not have a health plan relative to just 14% of the rural population. The problem persists in how healthcare facilities, hospitals, and emergency departments (the most probable option for the uninsured) are prepared to cope with the casualties of the pandemic.

• Health facilities become insignificant because the mechanisms are in place to ensure that pandemic influenza will not destroy health coverage and avoid the accelerated dumping of the deceased in communities (as in Philadelphia, which was compounded after World War I by hospital leaves). If medical staff excel in influenza, the length and intensity of the pandemic would be enhanced. During the 1918 pandemic in Philadelphia, "the city morgue had ten times as many bodies as coffins."

- A higher number of life insurance households will reduce the financial burden of missing the primary breadwinner of the household. Life insurance is a common benefit (positive to earnings); thus, low-income households are less likely than higher-income families to be covered by benefits.

- In the near term, urban quarantines will potentially damage companies. Employees will potentially be fired. Families without influenza touch can also suffer financial difficulties. The quarantine will be full to avoid spread (i.e., no operation beyond the home permitted). Partial quarantines, including shutting classrooms and hospitals but not mass transit and businesses, will do nothing to deter the outbreak of influenza like it did in Chicago, St. Louis, and Washington, D.C.

- Many businesses can experience sales losses of more than 50%. Some, such as health services and goods, could expand in business (unless there is complete quarantine). If the pandemic triggers a lack of workers, salaries for existing employees in certain sectors will rise temporarily. It is also less probable than in 1918, despite the improved productivity of staff today.

- Could we count on ity, state, and federal officials to assist in tackling a new pandemic? In the past, the administration has shown its failure to cope with crises (e.g., Hurricane Katrina). The consequences of a current influenza pandemic are likely to be mitigated by urban preparedness through public systems and clinics, charitable efforts (e.g., Red Cross), and private businesses, and conscientious acts of the community.

STRONGER PANDEMIC RESPONSE YIELDS BETTER ECONOMIC RECOVERY

For much of America in the closure phase to prevent the transmission of the SARS-CoV-2 outbreak, a controversy emerged as to whether the government should "reopen" commerce in order to reduce the economic effects of the pandemic. Yet in a recent report, co-authored by an MIT economist, the first factor that contributes to a better economic recovery is public safety.

Using data from the 1918-1919 flu pandemic in the US, the analysis showed that cities were behaving more aggressively to regulate social and public activities, and saw more economic activity during the restriction time.

Indeed, just ten days sooner than their predecessors, communities that introduced social-distance programs and other public safety initiatives reported a 5% rise in industrial workers since the 1923 pandemic. Likewise, 50 extra days of social isolation in a specific city is worth a 6.5% rise in manufacturing employment.

Emil Verner, an associate professor at the MIT Sloan School of Management and co-author of a new paper detailing the findings, said that "we find no evidence that cities that were more aggressive in the field of public health performed worse economically." In this respect, he noted, the notion of "trade-offs" between public health and economic activity does not remain a question of scrutiny; regions that are hardest hit by a pandemic are unable to recover their economic potential as quickly as locations which are more unaffected.

"This throws doubt about the notion of coping with the effects of an epidemic, on the one side, and economic development, on the other, because the pandemic itself becomes too harmful to the environment," Verner says.

The research, *Pandemics Depress the Economy, Public Health Interventions May not: Proof from the Grip of 1918*, was released as a working paper on 26 March by the Social Science Research Network. In addition to Verner, Sergio Correia, an economist with the USA, is the co-author. The Federal Reserve and the New York Federal Reserve Bank economist Stephen Luck is also a part of it.

Evaluating economic consequences

The three researchers reviewed US death rates in order to perform the study. Disease Control Centers (CDC), historical US economic info, The Census Bureau, and banking reports were collected by Mark D. Flood, a financial analyst, using a federal report entitled "*Currency Controller's Annual Reports.*"

As Verner says, scholars were urged to study the influenza pandemic of 1918-1919 and see if results might be taken from it in the present crisis.

"The purpose of the study is to concentrate on what the predicted economic effects of today's coronavirus would be and how the economic impacts of the public safety and social distancing measures that we see globally are to be mirrored," says Verner.

Scholars have recognized that the various applications of "non-pharmaceutical treatments" or social isolation mechanisms coincided with specific health effects in 1918 and 1919 across towns. As the pandemic struck, U.S. towns, such as St. Louis, shut down schools then there were others preferring grasp rather than shutdowns afterward, such as Philadelphia. This research applied the system to economic development.

Much as today, societal distancing steps at the time involved the closing of schools and theatres, collective prohibition, and restricted business practices.

"The non-pharmaceutical measures introduced in 1918 are quite close to those strategies utilized today to decrease SARS-CoV-2 distribution," says Verner.

Generally, the report shows that the pandemic had a significant economic effect. On the basis of state-level statistics, researchers witnessed an 18% decrease in manufacturing production until 1923, long after the last flu outbreak in 1919.

Nevertheless, in consideration of the impact in 43 towns, the researchers observed substantially different economic consequences correlated with specific policy lengths. Oakland, California; Denver,

Nebraska; Portland, Oregon, and Seattle, both of which practiced mutual distancing over 120 days in 1918, became the greatest cities in the country. Cities that developed social distinctions fewer than 60 days in 1918 and subsequently endured a development challenge included Philadelphia; St. Paul, Minnesota; and Lowell, Massachusetts.

"We note that the areas which were most severely impacted by the influenza pandemic in 1918 are undergoing a rapid and sustained downturn in many economic activity indicators, including mining, output, bank loans, and market sustainable inventory," Verner says.

Banking issues

So far as banking is concerned, the report also listed bank write-downs as an economic health measure, because "banks recognized losses in loans that households and businesses lost owing to economic uncertainty induced by the pandemic," said Verner.

Researchers noticed that the banking industry was struggling more in Albany, New York; Birmingham, Alabama; Boston; and Syracuse, New York — both of which were just within 60 days apart in 1918 – than in any other region of the world.

As stated by the writer, the economic difficulties after the grip pandemic of 1918-1919 limited industries 'capacity to produce products – however, the decline of jobs indicated that individuals still had fewer buying power.

"The proof we have in our report ... shows that both a supply-side concern and a demand-side question are triggered by the pandemic," Verner says.

As Verner readily recognizes, the structure of the US economy has changed from 1918-1919, with comparatively less output today and more service operations. The pandemic of 1918-1919 was also especially deadly for adults in the early working century, rendering its economic effects extremely serious. Nevertheless, analysts conclude that the complexities of the past pandemic will quickly be extended to our situation.

"The economic system is obviously different," Verner says. "Although we can not extrapolate from experience so explicitly, we should take certain lessons that might be important to us now." He stresses, first of all, "The economics of pandemics is distinct from the usual economy."

The Spanish Flu

HOW THE 1918 FLU PANDEMIC REVOLUTIONIZED PUBLIC HEALTH

Mass mortality has modified our way of thought and the position of the government in handling the disease.

Less than 100 years before in 1918, perhaps in the entire world of modern civilization, the planet witnessed the largest tidal wave of destruction since the Black Death. We name the Spanish flu this tidal wave, so several things changed as a consequence of most of the biggest movements in the world of public safety.

In the first decades of the 20th century, the planet was a very different location. Notably, when it came to education, there was no clear related philosophy. Many physicians either served for themselves or were supported by foundations or religious organizations in the developed world, and other patients had little connection to them.

Eugenics influenced public policy programs — such as citizenship laws. It was normal for wealthy leaders to regard laborers and the weak as lower groups of men, whose inherent degeneration predisposed them to sickness and deformity. Throughout the sometimes harsh living environments of the lower classes, these leaders did not try the triggers of disease: cramped tenements, lengthy working hours, poor health. The eugenicists claimed that although they became sickened and dying of typhus, cholera, and other monsters, it was their own guilt since they had little motivation for a decent standard of life. In the sense of an outbreak, public safety usually applied to a set of steps intended to defend the powerful from the contaminating impacts of the rabble.

During the beginning of 1918, the first outbreak of Spanish influenza struck. There was nothing about it. Yet flu is spread by the breath — by cough and sneezes, as we learn. This is extremely infectious and more readily distributed where individuals are placed in large densities, for example, in favelas or trenches. The first outbreak was comparatively moderate, not any different than common flu, but then in the fall of 1918, the second and worst period of the pandemic broke out; citizens could not imagine it to be the same disease. An alarmingly large number of people died — 25 times higher than in past influenza pandemics. While they reported the classic symptoms of flu — flare, sore throat, pain — they quickly turned blue in the face, and experienced respiratory difficulties, and even bleeding from their mouths and nose. If blue turned black, it was doubtful that they would survive. The congested lungs were actually too full of blood for air to absorb, and death typically resulted in hours or days. The second wave plummeted by the end of the year, but in early 1919 there was a third and final wave – moderate of virulence between the two.

By 1918, the flu was produced by a vaccine, but most physicians around the world believed that they had a bacterial illness. So they were almost totally helpless against the Spanish hold. They had no flu vaccine nor antibiotics that could have been effective against secondary bacterial infections (in the form of pneumonia), which killed the majority of their victims. Public health initiatives like quarantine and public meeting places could be successful, but often too late, even if implemented, as influenza was not reportable in 1918. This implied that physicians were not obligated to inform the authorities about events, which in turn meant that the pandemic did not come.

According to current estimates, the epidemic affected between 50 million to 100 million lives, or between 2.5 to 5% of the global population. World War I murdered 18 million men, and World War II destroyed about 60 million. Disease and mortality levels vary significantly across the planet for a variety of complicated cases that have been researched by epidemiologists. The less well-off endured more — albeit not for the purposes suggested by eugenicists — yet the wealthy were not spared.

The message that health officials learned from the tragedy was that it was no longer fair to punish or handle a person in isolation for the catching of an infectious disease. In the 1920s, several countries adopted the idea of socialized medicine — health insurance for all, given free of charge at the point of distribution. Russia became the first nation to set up a centralized public health program funded by state-run insurers and preceded by those in western Europe. The U.S. followed a separate direction, choosing employer-based benefits, but still taking steps to simplify post-influence healthcare.

In 1924 the Soviet Union introduced a viewpoint on the doctor of the future. He should "be willing to research the workplace and social factors that give rise to sickness and not just to treat the disease, but to recommend methods of avoiding it." That idea was slowly picked up across the globe. Public safety started to feel much like today.

Epidemiology — the analysis of trends, triggers, and consequences of illness — is the foundation of public safety and has been widely accepted as a discipline. Epidemiology needs evidence, and the gathering of health records has become increasingly comprehensive. In 1925, for example, every US state was participating in a regional program for monitoring diseases, and the lamentably lacking early warning infrastructure in 1918 took form. Ten years later, illustrating the growing concern of the authorities for the "baseline" wellbeing of the community, the people were subjected to the first nationwide wellbeing survey.

In the 1920s, several countries founded or revamped health ministries. The pandemic emerged either directly from cabinet councils with public safety officials or from lobbying for funding and resources from various authorities. However, it was always understood that public safety would be organized at the international level because infectious infections simply do not honor boundaries. In 1919, a foreign disease combat agency was established in Vienna, Austria, a forerunner to today's World Health Organization.

As the WHO came into being, eugenics became disgraced in 1946, and the statute of the independent body enshrined a completely fairly equitable commitment to health. He said: "The value of the highest practicable quality of safety is one of the basic freedoms of all citizens irrespective of ethnicity, faith, political opinion, economic or social circumstances." The possibility of influenza pandemics – three of which the WHO has encountered in their lives, and would certainly learn more – will not be abolished, but it will improve the way people are faced by it. And it emerged from an awareness that pandemics was a global epidemic, not a particular one.

MISCONCEPTIONS ABOUT THE 1918 FLU, THE 'GREATEST PANDEMIC IN HISTORY'

Yet pandemics have happened in the world before and worse. Also, remember the 1918 influenza pandemic, sometimes incorrectly referred to as 'Spanish flu,' which may contribute to false concerns as related cases occur in the future.

The 1918 pandemic officially killed between 50 and 100 million people, about 5% of the world's population. About a thousand individuals were tainted. The predilection of 1918 for the lives of otherly stable young people was especially noteworthy, as compared to children and the aged who typically struggle the most. Several media have called it the worst pandemic in history.

Over the last century, the 1918 influenza pandemic frequently became the topic of debate. There have been various theories produced by historians and scientists about its roots, its dissemination, and its implications. As a consequence, others haven't missed it.

By correcting these ten misunderstandings, everybody will fully grasp what occurred and tend to prevent potential events.

1. The pandemic originated in Spain

Nobody claims Spain's so-called "Spanish Disease."

This pandemic was possibly named after the First World War, which at the time was in full swing. The main countries in the war wanted to avoid helping their rivals, so influenza in Germany, Austria, France, the United Kingdom, and the United States was silenced. Neutral Spain, though, didn't have to hold the flu under wraps. This gave the false impression that Spain had the brunt of the disease.

Currently, the regional root of the flu remains debated up to today, while East Asia, Europe, and even Kansas have been proposed by theories.

2. The pandemic was the work of a 'super-virus.'

During the first six months of 1918, fever erupted exponentially, killing 25 million people. Some people were afraid for the end of humanity, and for a long time, the assumption was made that the flu strain was particularly lethal. However, recent studies have shown that the virus itself, though deadlier than other varieties, is not fundamentally different from the epidemics of other years.

Many of the high death rates may be due to crowds in military and urban settlements, and to poor nutrition and sanitation endured during the battle. It is now suspected that many of the deaths were due to the emergence of influenza-weakened bacterial pneumonia in the lungs.

3. The first wave of the pandemic was most lethal

In reality, the first wave of deaths from the pandemic was fairly small in the first half of 1918.

The largest mortality rates were recorded in the second phase, from October to December of that year. In the spring of 1919, a new wave became more devastating than the first but less than the second.

Researchers also assume that the significant rise in deaths in the second wave was induced by factors promoting the dissemination of a deadlier virus. Those with moderate cases often lived at home, while people with serious cases were clustered in clinics and camps with rapidly deadly virus spread.

4. The virus killed most people who were infected with it

The overwhelming number of citizens who developed influenza in 1918 still recovered. In total, national mortality rates among the infected did not reach 20%.

Death levels varied between various classes, though. In the USA, fatalities in Native Americans were especially large, possibly owing to lower levels of sensitivity to previous influenza strains. Entire tribal populations were, in several instances, wiped out. Of course, even a 20% death rate exceeds typical flu, killing less than 1% of the infected.

5. Therapies of the day had little impact on the disease

Throughout the 1918 flu, no clear anti-viral treatments were usable. This also remains true today, as the bulk of medical treatment for flu is meant to offer help instead of a cure for patients.

One theory indicates that aspirin toxicity may potentially be due to certain flu deaths. At the moment, medical experts prescribed large doses of aspirin of up to 30 grams a day. Today, the average healthy regular dosage will be about four grams. Huge doses of aspirin, including diarrhea, may have contributed to other effects of the pandemic.

Nevertheless, in certain areas around the world where medication was not so easily accessible, the mortality rate seemed to be similarly high, and the controversy persists.

6. The pandemic dominated the day's news

The magnitude of 1918 influenza, which culminated in a reduced profile in the newspapers, was underscored by public health authorities, law enforcement officers, and legislators. While believing that complete transparency might entice rivals throughout the battle, they needed to maintain public order to prevent hysteria.

Officials did, however, react. In several countries, quarantines were developed at the height of the pandemic. Many of them were required to restrict critical infrastructure, including police and security.

7. The pandemic changed the course of World War I

The result of World War I was impossible to improve with influenza since soldiers were nearly similarly impacted on both sides of the frontline.

However, there is no question that the course of the pandemic was heavily affected by the conflict. The influx of millions of troops produced perfect conditions for the creation of more violent virus strains and for its dissemination across the world.

8. Widespread immunization ended the pandemic

Immunization of influenza was not conducted in 1918, and the pandemic was not halted. Exposure to prior influenza strains could have given some security. For starters, soldiers who have served in the army for years have experienced lower mortality rates than new recruits.

Moreover, the rapidly mutating virus has probably evolved into less lethal strains over time. This is predicted by natural selection simulations. Because highly lethal strains rapidly destroy their host, they can't spread as easily as less deadly strains.

9. The genes of the virus have never been sequenced

In 2005, researchers reported that the 1918 influenza virus gene sequence had been effectively calculated. The virus was collected from the corpse of a flu survivor in Alaska's permafrost and reports of American soldiers who were also sick.

Two years later, virus-infected primates displayed the signs seen during the pandemic. Studies suggested the mortality of monkeys as the so-called "cytokine outbreak" overreacted to the virus in their immune systems. Scientists also suggest the same overreaction to the immune system related to a high death rate among relatively stable young adults in 1918.

10. The world is no better prepared today than it was in 1918

Every few decades, major epidemics exist, the current one is now on us.

Scientists now know much about isolating and treating a vast number of sick and suffering people, and physicians will administer antibiotics that did not occur in 1918 for fighting secondary bacterial infections. Contemporary medicine should incorporate vaccines and anti-viral medications to common sense activities, including social distancing and hand washing.

Viral epidemics will remain a frequent aspect of human life in the near future. As a business, we can only assume that we have grasped enough the great pandemic to quench any possible situation.

FLU PANDEMIC OF 1918: 5 LESSONS TAUGHT

Facts about the 1918 Spanish flu

- The 1918 flu epidemic killed 50 - 100 million people.

- The 1918 flu was an H1N1 virus (Swine Flu is an H1N1 virus also).

- In the Northern Hemisphere, in April, the first outbreak of the flu epidemic (as with swine flu) occurred.

- In four months, the first outbreak of Spanish flu destroyed 1-2 million men. More than 50 million people perished in the second wave.

Let us place it in perspective: more citizens are brought together than the entire Americans who perished in conflicts!! Then they waged other battles. That's more men than perished combined in BOTH world wars. The number of population worldwide is just over 300 million.

The epidemic of 1918 hit the globe in four months. This came before the age of aviation. If you can see, we can benefit a lot today from the outbreak of 1918, and it is from it that several pandemic preventive initiatives come. This requires just one infectious mutation, which may be greater than the influenza outbreak of 1918.

The government withheld details from the general population and promoted in its (mis)informational strategies a slogan "Do not be scared," which said, "You are protected when you take these measures." Which measures were you looking for?

Precautions

1) Public gatherings were restricted or prohibited.

2) Quarantine and isolation measures were used sporadically

3) Campaigns for awareness (actually used to reduce distrust through misinformation)

4) Deploying public health doctors and nurses

5) Ineffectual vaccinations.

6) Spitting banned

7) The use of a flu mask made compulsory for Mask Slackers with heavy fines.

Here And Now

How are we willing to refer right here and now? Sweet, we should self-impose 1 and 2, stop 3, and see 4 whether we choose to carry 5 (swine and avian flu vaccinations are minimal, so shop sterilizers so respiratory flu masks on hand. The CDC has created several nice detailed leaflets on the subject worth reading.

Shortages

According to a May *Time Magazine* report, there has been a major shortage of 3 m n95 flu masks (the most effective of the flu masks approved by the FDA) in the US. That is also valid in several other developing nations. The report notes that 119 million nasal flu masks are actually distributed in the United States. More than 1% of the approximate 30 billion n5 air flu masks expected to cover the United States adequately. The same deficiencies can still arise in all Tamiflu and Relenza influenza medications and vaccinations (which tend to have adverse effects). You should handle your body properly, even while experts disagree, it would surely not harm you to maintain approximately 100% of your immunity.

The problem is: who is going to be granted priority if and when the current outbreak becomes pandemic? It would be the only government official who has preferential access to a mask and injections of n95 respirator flu. If a pandemic of the second wave occurs, a scarcity may arise. The best way to ensure the exposure of producers now working at full capacity is to buy their own products until they are all bought by world governments. If you don't stay in a nation that makes goods such as the 3 m n95 vaccine flu mask or Tamiflu, you'll have much less opportunity, as these countries will have what they need for their own people.

The Spanish Flu

HOW THE 1918 SPANISH FLU PANDEMIC CHANGED THE NURSING PROFESSION: AN INTERVIEW

No medication, no vaccination, no antibiotics were necessary. Health experts reported that 500 million individuals across the globe – one-third of the world's population – were sick. Approximately 50 million people perished.

This lead to a variety of activities been held by the Science Schools and other schools at College of New Jersey in Ewing, including seminars, workshops, exhibits, a Flu-themed Escape the Space Tent, and a Flu Vaccine Clinic for students to receive their yearly vaccines.

Carole Kenner, a licensed nurse with a doctorate in medicine, who is now a professor at TCNJ's College at Medicine, Nutrition, and Exercise, recently spoke about Spanish flu and how it has contributed to drastic improvements in the nursing profession and healthcare business.

What was the Spanish flu? What happened?

It was a virus that at the point we understood nothing about. The first group, three of them, started in spring 1918 and really reached military installations, where citizens stayed in near communities. The normal trend takes place in the autumn, and the second phase started

How The 1918 Spanish Flu Pandemic Changed The Nursing Profession: An Interview

in the autumn of 1918. In the spring of 1919, the third wave happened. The reason it was named Spanish grippe is that Spain was more or less optimistic and not prone to the same restrictions as to what was happening. Among other nations, influenza happened, but you could not know anything about what was going on in a combat zone or military base.

Again, more people were exposed because of wartime conditions. Typically, two groups are particularly susceptible to whether you have an influenza outbreak or seasonal influenza: very young and very elderly people who have compromised their immune systems, too. The Spanish flu, though, infected 20, 30 and 40-year-olds.

We knew about it very little. We only realized we had an illness that destroyed people and that we wanted to be well. When it expanded — it came to the United States — everybody was scared. Somebody could be healthy one day, then dead the next night.

Nurses were stationed both in New Jersey and Philadelphia to serve in the service. A school was initially founded to train military nurses overseas. This indicated that many patients weren't there to look after the ill here. Often, the patients here got ill and died; six school pupils who offered to live and support perished. Family members often had to care for the sick.

Health authorities found a remedy. They chose to do a short training course for what they called a practical nurse in those days.

How did the nursing profession change as a result?

It was the origin of the clinical nurse section, as we know today and the licensed nurse. There were crowded clinics. We realized that not all could be educated at the same standard. The professional nurse had been qualified for three to six months and in the populations.

It unlocked doors for the nursing career at the same time. There was a tremendous need for specific skills. Before the pandemic, this was not known.

Grippe has raised the awareness of what nurses in these conditions might do. It has made it clear globally that nurses are the frontline care practitioners. They were more than surgeons. The importance of nursing became improved, and [...] its position in public welfare and culture became more noticeable.

More citizens were also drawn to the field. It has been repeated again and again in our past in moments of crisis, including even Spanish flu. Many thought, "I want to do it so nurses will save lives."

The health-care industry overall changed, as well?

Around the point, public service care was by the American Red Cross. This wasn't a caring for public welfare, as we know it now. They had to respond to such an enormous amount of people who were ill. It gave rise to the awareness that a better public health program was needed to respond to such disasters. People were frightened sufficiently to make them aware that they wanted help in groups that could lead to circumstances like this. Because this was a regional tragedy, the city needed to react to the local issue.

It reinforced and improved the public-health network. Over time, it has been a network in public safety and a warning mechanism. The slogan we use today is population-oriented safety and preparedness for disasters.

So the Spanish flu led to changes in how we respond to disasters?

Now, it is not always the first responders who come when we have catastrophes like flooding, tornadoes, hurricanes. There are social professionals from the Red Cross, public health facilities, outbreak management, and preventive centers. They respond in a more coordinated manner. You're referring to each other. They know where qualified people are and how, in a combat mission, they should send them.

We use social networking to extract details easily. For starters, I resided in Boston after the Boston Marathon bombing. We had marathon students who felt they should help with sprains and strains. We had no way to reach them after the attack since cell phone networks were blocked.

The Spanish Flu

Now we have these networks of warnings. Much as we get updates for power outages on our mobile phones, we are sending messages stating, "We need people to go to X." We have a network of posts. Cases go through a database such that you can continue to map the gaps and see when the person wants to be distributed.

All this arose out of the days, including the Spanish grip age, when we were absolutely overwhelmed.

Even with all these advances, what more needs to be done?

My fear now is that we are not raising enough support for our public health programs and divisions of public health. Such fields have been underfunded for some time and can, in some instances, be removed. There is always a chance of infections, be it infectious diseases or natural disasters. They need further technical programs. We will emphasize the collaborative approach in order to realize what we each bring to the table.

In the last few years, I've been on many flights where there's been a medical emergency. They can dial into the intercom for those with expertise with healthcare. Two or three of us will reply many times. They first ask, "I'm a nurse; my experience is ..." "I'm a doctor, my history is ..." And we know how to answer as a team.

In every occasion, an aged person felt tired and sweated. Three of us replied. My focus was on neonatal care. The other two were a thoracic and an oncologist. We thought, "Well, this is a wellness test. We can do this." His aircraft was overdue. He didn't have anything to feed. He became dehydrated. In a matter of minutes, we found it out. His glucose was tested. We gave him orange milk, and he just became well.

It's all those cases in which you have to bring together the squad that's available, know how to choose, know what the strengths are, and learn how to function effectively as a squad.

8 Things to know about pandemic influenza

There is still a possibility of pandemic influenza. A pandemic can occur if a new flu virus, which has previously not infected humans, spreads and causes serious illness.

Flu viruses are volatile – we can never be sure when or where the next pandemic will occur. However, another pandemic influenza is likely. The problem is not that we are going to get another pandemic in this industrialized planet, but when.

The WHO has issued a Global Influenza Strategy 2019-2030 to protect citizens all over the globe from this threat. The latest approach is WHO's most detailed and far-reaching influenza plan. The plan provides a process for the collective planning, prevention, and monitoring of influenza between WHO, countries, and stakeholders.

1. The influenza pandemic will arise – because we assume that another influenza pandemic will develop elsewhere. In 1918, the deadliest infectious epidemic in memory was the influenza pandemic in 1918. There has been three influenza pandemics since 1918-1957, 1968, and 2009 (H1N1). The possibility of a modern influenza virus spreading from livestock to humans that may contribute to a pandemic is possible and acts as a reminder that the next pandemic will always be planned.

2. Fluorine is now a significant safety threat. Seasonal influenza is a risk of illness across the year. Approximately 1 billion infections are reported per year, of which 3 to 5 million are serious, with 290 000 to 650 000 respiratory deaths associated with influenza worldwide. Reducing the effects of seasonal flu through increased management, detection, and tracking lets countries brace for a pandemic.

Call your commitment to influenza control and have your regular influenza injection. It is the safest way to avoid influenza.

3. They are more trained than we were – but still not trained sufficiently. Although a lot of research has been undertaken in preparing for a pandemic over the years, more needs to be done. It is important that all health facilities worldwide are equipped for influenza prevention and management.

We need safe and stable health services.

4. Since we are all related, cooperation is vital to the readiness of the planet for an influenza pandemic. The WHO, governments, and stakeholders must work together to achieve the goals of the plan and coordinate global and national influenza prevention, quick diagnosis, and reaction capacities.

5. Via this strategic strategy, the WHO and its collaborators will encourage the creation of improved global instruments for the prevention, diagnosis, control, and treatment of influenza. Such devices include improved vaccinations, antivirals, and therapies. The objective is to make them available to all nations.

6. The creation of stronger country capacity to track, adapt, avoid, and manage diseases and preparedness is the primary aim of this strategy. To do this, it calls for a tried and tested influenza system for every nation.

7. The price of preparedness will be much higher than the cost of major influenza outbreaks. A serious pandemic will lead to millions of deaths worldwide, with significant social and economic repercussions. The expense of planning for a pandemic is projected at less than USD 1 per person per year, less than 1% of the expected cost of reacting to a pandemic.

8. Investing in influenza prevention, control, and preparedness initiatives would allow countries to reap gains beyond influenza through the overall improvement of their health care systems. Countries should connect their influenza activities with other national and global health and safety initiatives.

CONCLUSION

The 1918 influenza was the deadliest outbreak in American memory. Hundreds of thousands perished, and the extremely infectious influenza virus was transmitted by millions. Analysis into the pandemic of 1918 also centered on the possibility of a future influenza pandemic as a basic blueprint for the likely effects of a new influenza epidemic in the United States. Furthermore, given the magnitude of influenza in 1918, very few works have been done into the economic consequences of the pandemic. In this article, the economic impact of the influenza pandemic of 1918 was addressed and evaluated based on available data and analysis. The flu of 1918 was short-lived and had "a lasting effect not on societies, but on the atoms of human society – on individuals." Although civilization as a whole quickly healed from the flu in 1918, people affected by the flu saw their lives forever altered. With our highly mobile and linked population, given advances in health care in the past 90 years, any potential pandemics of influenza will be more severe and potentially more virulent than the 1918 influenza. Learning from experience might maybe serve to reduce the impact of any potential pandemic. Of necessity, it needs coordination and preparation at both levels of government and the private sector to avert a pandemic. Unfortunately, the 2005 study reveals that the United States is not preparing for a pandemic of influenza.

Although federal, state, and local governments in the US have begun to focus in recent years on preparedness, progress has been slow, especially at the local government level. There's been poor coordination at various governments' levels in response to the past disaster. If people choose governments to prevent an influenza epidemic, policy preparation, and the ability to protect citizens from a pandemic should be a matter of concern. Perhaps the best way to protect citizens in the case of a potential flu pandemic is public education about flu prevention, greater reliance on charity groups and charitable organizations, and a dose of personal responsibility.

Conclusion

Do Not Go Yet; One Last Thing To Do

If you enjoyed this book or found it useful, I'd be very grateful if you'd post a short review on Amazon. Your support does make a difference, and I read all the reviews personally so I can get your feedback and make this book even better.

Thanks again for your support!

www.ingramcontent.com/pod-product-compliance
Lightning Source LLC
Chambersburg PA
CBHW071125240526
45465CB00024B/1201